FEELING SEXY IN MY NEW BODY!

A QUICK GUIDE OF PRACTICAL FAT-LOSS STRATEGIES FOR PEOPLE WHO ARE STRUGGLING TO LOSE WEIGHT

EDDIE E. ERICKSON

This book is dedicated to all of the millions of people out there struggling to lose weight.

TABLE OF CONTENTS

ACKNOWLEDGEMENTS

I would like to thank my family and friends for encouraging me while writing this book and all of the editors and other helpful people at Amazon and CreateSpace who made this book possible.

INTRODUCTION

A journey of a thousand miles begins with a single step. —Chinese Proverb

Congratulations on taking the first step toward losing fat, improving your health and energy, and creating the slim, new you. This book is full of practical and proven strategies for successful fat loss. I decided to write this book because I see so many people struggling to lose weight. Obviously, there is a lot of confusion out there, because the obesity epidemic has been getting worse for decades and is now exploding. It's not just an American problem anymore. It's now becoming a worldwide problem. So many people are confused about what to eat, what not to eat, what really works, and how to actually lose fat and keep it off. I have been into bodybuilding for 33 years. I aim to cut through all the confusion and nonsense out there and tell you exactly what really does work.

Maybe you woke up one day, looked in the mirror, and realized that you had gained 10, 20, 50, 100, or more pounds, and you have no idea how to get rid of the fat. Are you tired of trying to find clothes that fit well? Are you tired of hauling all that excess weight around? Are you tired of being tired? Maybe you have tried countless fad diets and weight-loss supplements, and nothing worked. You might be one of those millions of people who do try to exercise and eat right, but the scale never budges. In this book, I explain why that scale never budges and what you can do about it to finally get the results you want! Are you ready to get serious and finally get into shape? Are you disgusted with the flab and ready to take action? Let me help you do an "extreme makeover" on yourself. Let's create the slim, new you!

MY STORY

I can sympathize with other people who have gained weight. I understand how the pounds can sneak up on you. I woke up one day at age 42 and realized that I had gained 30 pounds of fat. Astonishingly, I didn't even realize that I had gained all that fat until I saw a picture of myself on the beach in Mexico. Was that really me? I could not believe it. Sure, my pants had got a bit tighter, but I had not paid much attention to that, and I had not weighed myself in a long time. I have been an athlete and into fitness and noncompetitive bodybuilding for most of my life. As I reached my early 40s, my metabolism apparently slowed down, which seems to happen to a lot of people and is supposedly normal as we age. I had taken a big layoff from my normal routine to travel and to pursue other interests. I had slacked off on my exercise routine and let my normal, healthy diet slip a bit. I was eating way too many fattening foods and not exercising much at all. If a "health nut" athlete like me could pack on the fat, it could happen to anybody. I had never let myself get that heavy before. I immediately took action and burned off those 30 pounds of fat over a period of about four months. Years later, I am proud to say that I maintained the weight loss, and I am in close to the best shape of my life at age 47. I would like to share my 33 years of bodybuilding experience and knowledge with you to help you reach your weight-loss goals in the fastest time possible.

THE GOOD NEWS

The good news is that I can help you to lose fat and feel and look better. I have sorted through mountains of information and research to figure out what really works and what doesn't work. In addition to successfully losing weight myself, I have also studied other people who have done the same. If you follow my program, I promise you that you will have more energy, you will feel better, look better, and be healthier, and you will shed fat. It's not easy, but the rewards are well worth it. It takes patience, work, and dedication. Chances are good that you didn't gain 20, 50, or 100 pounds overnight, so don't expect to lose it overnight either. If it were easy to lose weight and get into shape, everyone would have a great body. In this book, I try to cut through all the confusion and clutter. I have condensed volumes of information down into something that is easy and manageable to read and understand. But best of all, this information will work for you if you apply it consistently.

CONSULTING YOUR DOCTOR

Always consult your doctor before starting a weight-loss plan, and make sure that it is OK for you to do so. Knowing your blood pressure, blood sugar, cholesterol levels, triglycerides, C-reactive protein, and resting heart rate can be very eye-opening. Watching these numbers improve as you eat right and get into shape can be just as motivating as watching our weight drop!

LET'S TAKE ACTION AND GET STARTED!

In this book I explain how and why we gain weight, how to lose fat, how to get motivated and energized, how to get results, and how to keep the fat off once you have lost it. I explain what foods are making us heavy, what role leptin plays, exactly what foods we should be eating for good health and energy, and what role our self-image plays in our fat-loss efforts. I explain the role of our metabolisms and tell you how to speed up yours. I give you some practical advice to help you reach your weight loss goals in record time. This book can help you to melt the fat off, increase your energy, improve your appearance, and create a slim, new you. If you are ready, let's get started!

Chapter 1:

How Did We Gain All This Weight?

The secret of getting ahead is getting started. —Mark Twain

There are hundreds of millions of people out there struggling to lose weight. The weight-loss industry is a multi-billion-dollar industry. There are countless fad diets, low-glycemic diets, low-carb diets, and starvation diets on the market. There are diet pills, drugs, drinks, and supplements. Some people have taken the drastic step of having gastric bypass surgery. Other people have simply thrown in the towel and given up on trying to lose weight. There are others who have lost weight and gained it all back and then some. So there is obviously a lot of confusion about what works in terms of weight loss and what doesn't work. My goal for this book is to clear up the confusion and make it very obvious as to what really works for weight loss so you can create the body that you want.

The obesity epidemic continues to get worse every year.

The following statistics are from the World Health Organization:

* Worldwide obesity has about doubled since 1980.
* There are now over 1 billion overweight adults in the world.
* Without action, there will be about 1.5 billion overweight adults by 2015.
* Roughly 300 million people are clinically obese in the world.

These statistics are from the Centers for Disease Control (CDC):

* In America today, about 69% of the population is overweight.
* About one-third of US adults are obese (33.8%).
* In 2008, medical costs associated with obesity were estimated at $147 BILLION.
* The problem is clearly getting worse. Consider that in 1985, no state in the US had more than 20% obesity rates. By 2009, nine states had obesity rates greater than 30%.

The American Journal of Preventative Medicine says this:

* Obesity has now become an equal, if not greater, contributor to disease than smoking.[1]

THE OBESITY EPIDEMIC AMONG CHILDREN

The percentage of children who are overweight or obese is higher than ever before. Globally, an estimated 10% of school-aged children between the ages of 5 and 17 years old are overweight or obese. Notice from the chart below that the prevalence of obesity among children and teens in America has more than quadrupled since 1970. Currently, about one out of five children are obese. Children and adolescents who are overweight tend to grow into overweight adults.

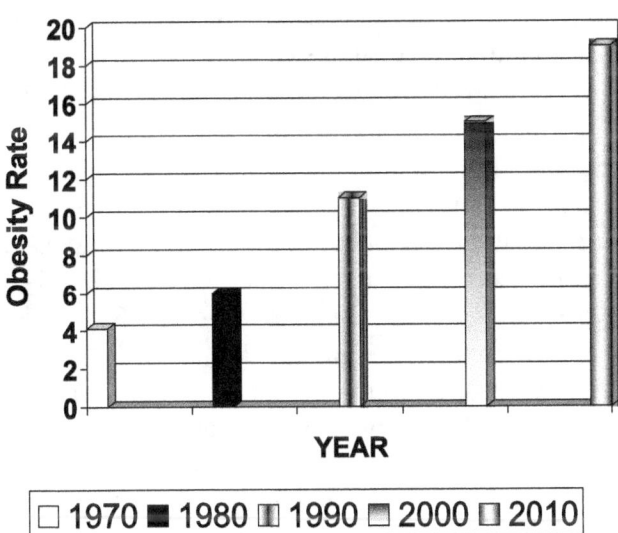

Obesity Rate Among US Children and Teens Ages 6 - 19

□ 1970 ■ 1980 ▥ 1990 ▨ 2000 ▢ 2010

Source: Centers for Disease Control

3

WHAT IS CAUSING THE OBESITY EPIDEMIC IN AMERICA?

A key to losing weight is first understanding what is driving the obesity epidemic and how we likely gained weight in the first place. The obesity epidemic is a disturbing but interesting phenomenon that has sparked a heated debate about what is actually causing it, but here are some possible explanations:

(1) Our population is becoming more sedentary.

We don't get as much exercise as our ancestors did. We are becoming more sedentary due to the invention of the automobile, other modern conveniences, and entertainment media. For most of human history, people walked for miles every day while hunting and gathering. All of a sudden, relatively speaking, we have automobiles and other modern conveniences. Most people no longer do much walking. Many people work in sedentary jobs instead of doing the physically demanding work of our ancestors. Instead of being outdoors playing and getting exercise, American children and teens 8–18 years of age now spend an average of 7.5 hours a day using entertainment media, including TV, computers, video games, cell phones, and movies. Of those 7.5 hours, about 4.5 hours is spent watching TV.[2] Overweight children tend to become overweight adults. Once adults get home from sedentary jobs, it is so easy and tempting to just relax in front of the TV or surf the Internet instead of exercising.

(2) We are consuming more calories. We have

become a fast-food nation.

Junk food is plentiful, and billions of dollars are spent annually on advertising it. There has been an explosion of fast-food restaurants across America. One estimate states that there are now 160,000 fast-food restaurants that serve over 50 million Americans daily and generate annual sales of about $65 billion. Most of these fast-food places serve high-calorie foods that are full of saturated and trans fats as well as salt and processed sugar. Temptation is everywhere. Our convenience stores and supermarkets are stocked full of unhealthy, energy-dense, processed junk. It seems that we can't go anywhere without being tempted with junk food. Fast-food restaurants are now popping up all over the rest of the world. Other countries with relatively lean populations are now becoming more westernized and gaining weight.

(3) We are eating a diet high in refined fructose, which leads to leptin resistance. (I explain this later in the chapter).

THE COUNTRIES WITH HIGHEST AND LOWEST RATES OF OBESITY IN THE WORLD

The tiny island country of Nauru has the highest obesity rate in the world. About 95% of the population of Nauru is overweight, and about 80% are obese. Nauru also has the highest rate of type 2 diabetes in the world. Kidney and heart disease are common. The average life span there is now under age 50. Due to little arable land, most of the local diet consists of imported, Western food such as lunch meat, corned beef and other canned meats, sugar snacks, high-fructose soda, and other processed foods. The most popular dish is fried chicken and cola. Fruit and vegetables are almost nonexistent in the stores because they are way too expensive to import. The local economy used to rely on the phosphate mines, but the mines are now depleted and the local economy is now in the dumps. There are few other resources. The lifestyle in Nauru is very laid-back and sedentary. Obesity was once seen as a sign of wealth and power in Nauru, but now the government is trying to encourage exercise and weight loss.[3]

In sharp contrast to the people of Nauru, the Japanese have one of the lowest obesity rates in the world at around 3%. That is about 10 times lower than in the United States. The Japanese also have the highest life expectancy in the world (83.5 years). What are the secrets of the Japanese? The staple food in Japan is Japonica (Japanese rice). It is a type of white rice that retains all the health benefits of brown rice. Japan is a vegetable-crazed nation. Cabbage, broccoli, and spinach are popular. Fishing is a big part of the economy. Consequently, the Japanese diet is extremely high in fish and other seafood. Grilled fish is common for breakfast. Beef, chicken, and pork are eaten, but they are treated as condiments rather than the main course of the meal. Fatty dairy products and white bread are not a big part of the diet. Fresh fruit is the preferred dessert. The Japanese don't snack on processed junk and colas like we do here in America. They do have vending machines, but the machines are stocked full of unsweetened tea and coffee beverages. Green tea is popular, and it is consumed instead of high-fructose soda. They do a tremendous amount of walking. They usually don't drive to work because parking is scarce and expensive. So, they either take the trains, bike, or walk to work. There are bicycles everywhere in Japan.[4]

OBESITY RATES OF 3 COUNTRIES

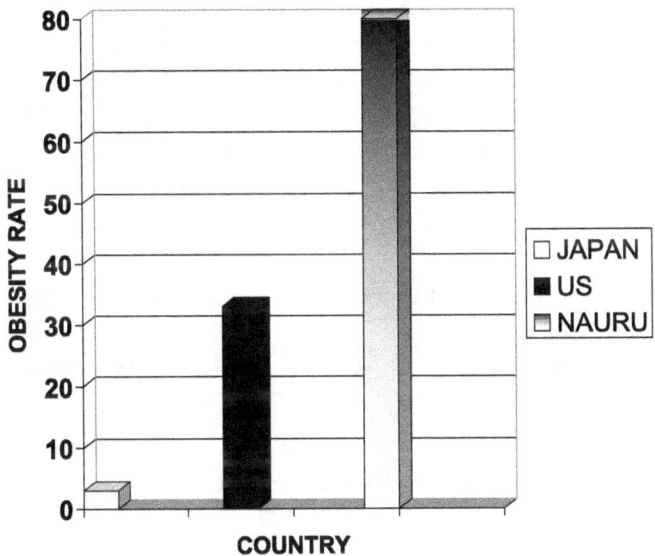

Source: World Health Organization

In summary, the people of Nauru are eating a lot of imported, high-calorie, processed junk and getting very little exercise. They hardly eat any fruit or vegetables at all. The Japanese are eating a lot of low-calorie rice, fish, fruit, and vegetables. The Japanese do a lot of walking and biking, and they avoid processed "empty-calorie" junk. Speaking of calories, what exactly is a calorie, and why is it so important?

DEFINING A CALORIE

A calorie is a unit of energy derived from food. You burn calories (energy) just getting through the day. Our metabolisms are constantly burning calories. You burn calories continually just from sleeping, lounging around the house, doing routine chores, or working in the office. But if you consume more calories in a day than you burn up, all the excess calories are stored as fat.

One pound of excess weight equals 3,500 calories. Ten pounds of excess weight is equal to 35,000 calories. If you want to lose weight, you have to cut the number of calories you consume and/or increase the number of calories you burn.

We **GAIN** weight when we consume more calories than we burn.
We **LOSE** weight when we burn more calories than consume.
We **MAINTAIN** our weight when our calorie consumption equals our calorie burn.

FOOD VOLUME AND FEELING SATISFIED

The feeling of fullness and satisfaction after a meal is actually determined by the volume and weight of the food in the stomach and not necessarily by the amount of calories in the food. Fruits and vegetables are considered to be low-density foods because they have a very few calories stored in a relatively large weight and volume. Foods with a lot of fat and/or processed sugar are considered to be high-density foods because they store a large amount of calories in a relatively small amount of space. For example, consider the following very large salad and drink:

1 cup of spinach: 14 calories
1/2 cup of broccoli: 12 calories
1/2 cup of cucumbers: 7 calories
1/2 cup of mushrooms: 9 calories
1/2 large tomato: 12 calories
1/2 cup carrots: 24 calories
1 clove of garlic: 4 calories
Sprinkle of lemon pepper: 0 calories
1 tbsp of fat-free Italian dressing: 20 calories
1 large iced tea with lemon slice: 0 calories

The grand total for the above meal is only 102 calories! Think of the volume that all of that food would take up in your stomach. You could eat a very large portion and walk away feeling full and satisfied for hours. Fruits and vegetables are full of volume and fiber, which takes a long time to digest and keeps you full. For comparison, consider some high-density foods:

Mayonnaise (1 tbsp): 90 calories
Shortening (1 tbsp): 113 calories
Lard (1 tbsp): 115 calories
Coconut oil (1 tbsp): 125 calories
Sausage (3 links): 132 calories
Ranch dressing (1 tbsp): 148 calories
Whole milk (1 cup): 150 calories
Cola (12 ounces): 160 calories
Peanut butter w/salt (1 tbsp): 188 calories
Chocolate cake (1 slice): 235 calories
Candy bar (2 ounces): 271 calories
Ice cream (1 cup): 290 calories
Fast-food bacon cheeseburger: 1080 calories

Just one tiny tablespoon full of mayonnaise has about the same amount of calories as that huge salad and iced tea. Notice that ranch dressing has a whopping 148 calories in just one tablespoon. If you happen to drench your salad in ranch dressing like a lot of people, you might be looking at an extra 500 calories! *One of the keys to weight loss is just cutting down on high-density foods and replacing them with low-density foods. You could gorge on fruits and vegetables all day long, stay full, and actually consume very few calories.*

Low-density vs. High-density foods

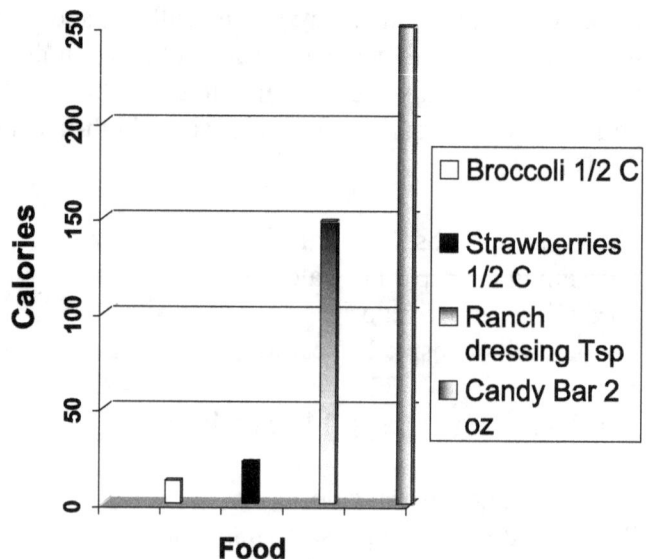

Source: Nutrition Almanac

CUTTING CALORIES IS THE OBVIOUS SOLUTION

Cutting calories to lose weight is so obvious that millions of people overlook it or refuse to believe it. But if you really think about it, it makes perfect sense. A calorie is a measurement of the amount of energy contained in food. Getting rid of excess fat is a matter of simple mathematics. Consume fewer calories than you expend, and your body has NO CHOICE but to burn stored energy to make up the energy difference!

Think of your checking account at the bank. If your withdrawals equal your deposits, your cash balance stays the same. If you withdraw more money than you deposit, your cash balance shrinks. It's simple math. If your cash deposits (calories) are greater than your cash withdrawals (calorie expenditure), your cash balance (waistline) grows.

So, if cutting calories is the way to lose weight, why not just go on a total starvation diet? Well, for one thing, you lose a lot of muscle when you do that. The proportion of muscle loss to fat loss when you fast is 60% to 40%. You are actually losing more muscle than fat when you fast. The second problem with a total starvation diet is that your body needs a certain amount of daily nutrients such as protein, carbohydrates, fats, vitamins, and minerals to function properly. You would quickly develop several nutritional deficiencies on a total starvation diet. The third problem with a total starvation diet is that your body goes into "famine mode" because it thinks that you are starving (which is actually the case), so your metabolism slows way down.

The answer is to eat a nutritious, balanced, low-calorie diet that provides all of the necessary nutrients for your body to be healthy and to function properly. This means making every calorie count. Never eat anything that does not satisfy your nutritional needs. Eliminate empty-calorie foods and drinks that provide a lot of calories but no nutritional value. Cut down on foods that contain high-calorie, unhealthy saturated fat, and totally eliminate foods that contain deadly trans fat. I will explain this in detail in the next chapter.

LOW CARB? LOW FAT? LATEST RESEARCH SAYS CALORIES COUNT MORE!

A 2004–2007 study led by the Harvard School of Public Health and Pennington Biomedical Research Center found that the key to losing weight comes down to a basic rule: calories in, calories out.[5] In other words, if you burn more calories than you consume, you lose weight. Likewise, if you eat more calories than you burn, you gain weight.

In the study, researchers randomly assigned 811 overweight adults to one of four diets, each of which contained different levels of fat, protein, and carbohydrates. The diets were twists on commercial plans. The four diets in the study contained healthy fats; were high in whole grains, fruits, and vegetables; and were low in cholesterol. Each dieter was required to slash a modest 750 calories a day from their weight maintenance level as determined by the scientists, perform only 90 minutes of modest exercise per week, keep a food diary, and meet regularly with diet counselors to chart their progress.

The results were as follows: there was no winner among the different diets. People had lost an average of 13 pounds at six months. After two years, dieters who stuck with it and met regularly with the counselors had lost and average of 22 pounds, regardless of which diet they followed. Remember, that was with just very moderate exercise. The lesson here is that there was no significant difference with different combinations of protein, carbs, and fats. What really mattered was calorie reduction and exercise.

Notice that the above diets contained only fruit and complex carbohydrates and no processed empty-calorie carbohydrates. There was a good reason for that, which I will explain in the next chapter.

Fat-loss strategy #1: Reduce calories for weight loss, but also eat a nutritious, well-balanced diet.

HOW DO WE CUT CALORIES?

(1) Eat less.

Forget liposuction—try lip obstruction! — Unknown

(2) Eat healthier.

Replace the empty-calorie foods that contain a lot of calories but few nutrients with nutrient-dense foods that contain fewer calories. For example, replace desserts with sweet fruits like strawberries and oranges. Cut down on calorie-dense foods that cause health problems.

LEPTIN RESISTANCE MAY PLAY A ROLE IN WEIGHT GAIN

Leptin is a hormone that plays a role in regulating energy intake and expenditure, appetite, and metabolism. Leptin signals to the brain that the body has had enough to eat, producing a feeling of fullness. The effects of leptin were observed in 1950 while studying morbidly obese mice that arose at random within a mouse colony. It was discovered that the obese mice had mutations in the "ob/ob" or "db/db" genes. These genes regulate leptin. Leptin itself was discovered in 1994. When obese mice with the "ob/ob" gene mutation are injected with leptin, they lose fat and return to their normal body weights.[6] However, the leptin injection does not work on the mice with the "db/db" gene mutation. A very tiny group of humans have mutations in the leptin gene that leads to a constant desire for food, resulting in morbid obesity. Human injections of leptin only appear to work for these very rare, obese individuals who produce zero leptin.

Other people have enough leptin but are simply resistant to the effects of leptin. Obese individuals generally have unusually high concentrations of leptin circulating in their bodies.[7] These individuals are resistant to the effects of leptin, just like type 2 diabetics are resistant to the effects of insulin. For whatever reason, the brain is just not getting the leptin signal. It is known that leptin levels in the body are proportional to body fat since leptin is produced by fat tissue. *Interestingly, leptin resistance easily arises in lab animals when they are given unlimited access to energy-dense foods!*[8] The leptin resistance is reversed when the animals are put back on low-density chow.[9] Some scientists say that this may be a built-in evolutionary advantage to store energy during times of feast. Animals have always been subject to frequent famines, and so were our human ancestors.

What actually causes leptin resistance? Leptin resistance arises from impaired leptin transport across the blood-brain barrier. An important study by William Banks, Alan Coon, et al., which was published by the American Diabetes Foundation, showed that elevated triglycerides in the blood are a main cause of leptin resistance.[10] Therefore, reducing triglycerides in the blood is a way to enhance transport of leptin across the blood-brain barrier. Total starvation also causes decreased transport of leptin across the blood-brain barrier. The evolutionary advantage of decreased leptin during times of starvation is very obvious. Decreased leptin means increased hunger and a greater drive to find food. So, the bottom line is that we want to reduce our triglycerides and never go on a total starvation diet for weight loss.

What exactly are triglycerides and how do we reduce them? In the simplest terms, triglycerides are fat in the blood. Any excess calories from carbohydrates or fat are converted into triglycerides. High levels are linked to atherosclerosis, heart disease, and stroke. We can reduce triglycerides by exercising, losing weight, and reducing our consumption of refined fructose, saturated fat, trans fat, alcohol, and cholesterol. Eating omega-3 fatty acids from fish and flax oil and supplementing with the amino acid L-carnitine also have been shown to lower triglyceride levels.

So it seems that leptin resistance is a vicious cycle. The unlimited access of energy-dense foods increases triglycerides and eventually causes leptin resistance in the lab animals, so they stay hungry and never quit eating. They become morbidly obese because the brain is no longer getting the "I'm full" signal from the body. *Now remember that the leptin resistance was reversed in the lab animals when they were put back on a normal diet of low-density chow. It seems to me that the same results may apply to humans.*

FRUCTOSE, LEPTIN, AND OBESITY

For thousands of years, humans consumed relatively small amounts of naturally occurring fructose from fresh fruits. Now we have high-fructose corn syrup (HFCS) and other high-fructose sweeteners added to soft drinks, juice beverages, packaged foods, cereals, and baked goods. In 1970, per capita consumption of HFCS in America was .5 lb/year, and by 1997 it was 43 lbs/year![11] Interestingly, we have seen a huge explosion in obesity since 1970. The use of HFCS has declined somewhat since 2000. Apparently, word is getting out that HFCS might be bad for us. What are some of the problems with consuming large amounts of HFCS and other types of refined fructose? Studies have shown that dietary refined fructose increases triglycerides (TG) and reduces circulating leptin.[12] Recall that high TG levels are a main cause of leptin resistance and also atherosclerosis.

Per Capita Consumption of HFCS in US

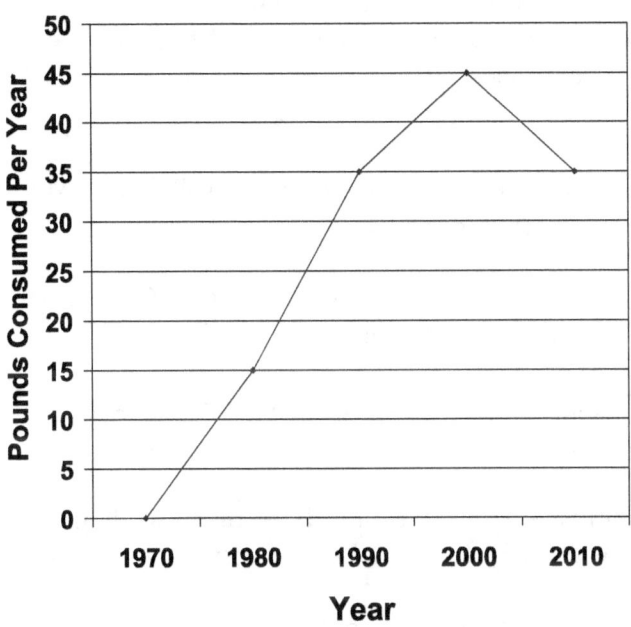

Source: USDA

In a study by Alexandra Shapiro, Wei Mu, Carlos Roncal, et al. at the University of Florida, the researchers performed an experiment on two groups of rats.[13] All of the rats ate the same diet except that one group consumed a lot of fructose while the other group received zero fructose. The study went on for six months. At the end of the study, there was no significant difference in bodyweight between the two groups of rats. *However, the high-fructose rats had developed very high triglyceride (TG) levels and had become leptin resistant.* The researchers then fed both groups of rats a high-calorie, high-fat diet. They found that the high-fructose, leptin resistant rats ate more and gained much more weight than the leptin-responsive animals. The study shows that a high refined-fructose diet can eventually lead to leptin resistance and a big weight gain when combined with a calorie-dense diet.

Refined-fructose---->High triglyceride (TG) levels--------->Leptin resistance

Leptin resistance-->Constant hunger-->Calorie-dense diet-->Big weight gain

Reduce TG's----->Leptin reaches brain----->Less hunger------->Eat fewer calories----->Fat loss

Fat loss--->Lower TG levels--->Increased leptin sensitivity by brain--->Less hunger

     In summary, avoid junk foods that are full of high-fructose corn syrup and other refined sweeteners because it could possibly lead to high triglyceride levels and leptin resistance.

     What other foods should we avoid? That is the subject of the next chapter.

CHAPTER 2:

WHAT FOODS TO AVOID

If hunger is not the problem, then eating is not the solution. —Anonymous

In this chapter, I explain exactly what foods to avoid if we want to lose weight, and why these foods are bad for us.

CARBOHYDRATES EXPLAINED

All sugars and starches are converted by the body into a simple sugar called glucose. Some of the glucose is used as fuel by the body. A small portion of the glucose is converted into glycogen by the body and stored in the liver and muscles for future energy needs. Any excess glucose calories are converted into fat and stored throughout the body as a reserve source of energy.[14] The fat storage is a survival mechanism that is great in times of famine but not so great in the modern world. Remember: fat is just stored energy.

What happens when we exercise? When we exercise, the fat reserves are converted back into glucose and used for energy, and weight-loss results.

With the popularity of low-carb diets, many people are afraid to eat any carbs at all, but it is important to distinguish between the processed (bad) carbs and the healthy (good) carbs.

AVOID PROCESSED CARBOHYDRATE FOODS

So, given what we now know about processed fructose, it makes sense to avoid processed carbohydrate foods that are very often full of high-fructose corn syrup and other forms of processed fructose. Processed carbs are the empty calories that I have been referring to. Processed carbohydrates are the bad carbs. These are foods with poor nutritional profiles. Most processed carb foods are a quick source of energy because they are rapidly digested and converted into glucose. Most foods that are high in processed carbohydrates contain few nutrients but a lot of calories. These are empty-calorie foods that lack fiber and pass into the bloodstream very quickly. Table sugar and many other processed carbs can alter your mood, lead to compulsive eating, and cause wild swings in your insulin and blood-sugar levels. Sometimes these wild mood swings are very obvious in children (and some adults) who consume a lot of candy. They experience a "sugar rush" along with an energy surge and hyperactivity, but crash a short time later.

Remember that we are trying to cut unnecessary calories from our diets to lose weight. We are trying to make every calorie count, so it makes good sense to eliminate foods that have a lot of calories but little nutritional value.

Sugar is a type of bodily fuel, yes, but your body runs about as well on it as a car would. —V.L. Allineare

According to the World Health Organization,

processed carbs are a leading factor in the obesity epidemic.

Some examples of empty-calorie, processed carbohydrates include:

* Soft drinks
* Sweetened fruit drinks
* Candy
* Jellies and jams
* Maple syrup
* Molasses
* Sugar cereals
* Most baked goods
* Dressings
* High-fructose corn syrup
* High-fructose packaged goods
* Table sugar
* Brown sugar
* White flour products
* Most desserts
* White bread
* White pasta

    *** **NOTE**: I am realistic and realize that it is almost impossible to avoid all processed carbohydrates and sweeteners. My own preference in this area is HONEY, which is all natural and actually packed full of several vitamins and minerals.

WHAT IS THE GLYCEMIC INDEX, AND IS IT RELEVANT?

    The glycemic index (GI) is a measure of the short-term effects of carbohydrates on blood-sugar levels. Carbs that digest quickly and release glucose quickly into the bloodstream have high GI values. When glucose rises quickly, this causes a spike in insulin, which stabilizes blood glucose. Insulin temporarily stops the use of fat as an energy source. Carbs that digest slowly and release glucose slowly have low GI values. Lower GI usually equates to a lower insulin spike by the body and supposedly, less fat storage. The GI tells us the effect on blood sugar from eating exactly 50 grams of a carbohydrate. The problem is that a normal serving of various foods is usually not exactly 50 grams, which makes it difficult to compare foods. So to solve that problem, the glycemic load index was developed.

The glycemic load (GL) tells us the short-term effects on blood-glucose levels from a **typical serving** of any particular food. Many modern diets rely on the GL. But there are a few problems with the GI and GL theory. For example, a junk food like chocolate cake has a relatively low GL of 20 and a deep-fried donut has a low GL of 15, while white rice has a very high GL of 36.[15] *White rice is a staple food in many countries with very low rates of diabetes and obesity.* As you might recall, white rice is a staple food of the Japanese diet, and the Japanese are among the leanest people in the world. Another problem with the GL theory is that when you mix foods together in a meal, the GL values get "averaged out" and become blurred. For example, if you mixed a high-GL food with a medium-GL food and two low-GL foods, would you still get an insulin spike? The answer can get complicated. Protein and fat tend to lower the glycemic index of a meal. The total amount of carbohydrates in a meal seems to be a stronger predictor of blood glucose than GI.

What does the American Diabetes Association say about the GI?

Research shows that both the amount and the type of carbohydrate in food affect blood glucose levels. Studies also show that the total amount of carbohydrate in food, in general, is a stronger predictor of blood glucose response than the GI. Based on the research, for most people with diabetes, the first tool for managing blood glucose is some type of carbohydrate counting. Balancing total carbohydrate intake with physical activity and diabetes pills or insulin is the key to managing blood glucose levels. Because the type of carbohydrate does have an affect on blood glucose, using the GI may be helpful in "fine-tuning" blood glucose management. In other words, combined with carbohydrate counting, it may provide an additional benefit for achieving blood glucose goals for individuals who can and want to put extra effort into monitoring their food choices.[16]

The bottom line is that we want to avoid empty-calorie carbohydrates for weight loss because they supply a lot of processed fructose and calories, and very little nutritional value; and because the total amount of carbs in a food is a greater predictor of glucose response than GI. We want to make every calorie count. Cutting down on processed carbs makes a lot of sense if you have diabetes and/or you are trying to lose weight.

Complex carbs and fruit, however, are a whole different ball game. Complex carbs and fruit are nutrient dense. Fruit and vegetables are water dense. Water has zero calories. Complex carbs contain a lot of fiber, digest slowly, and very slowly release glucose throughout the day. I explain complex carbs in detail in the next chapter.

Fat-loss strategy #2: Cut down on processed carbohydrates, especially refined fructose. Make every calorie count.

ENERGY-DENSE, CALORIE-DENSE FOODS

These are foods that are high in saturated fat and/or trans fat.

FATS: THE GOOD, THE BAD, AND THE UGLY

Fats are the most concentrated source of energy in the diet. Fats contain about twice the amount of calories and energy per gram as the same amount of proteins or carbohydrates. Excessive amounts of fat in the diet may lead to obesity if more calories are consumed than needed by the body. However, some fat is needed in the diet for good health. Fats act as carriers for the fat-soluble vitamins A, D, E, and K. Fat is also needed to keep the skin healthy and youthful by preventing dryness. Most nutritionists recommend a daily intake of fat that provides 25–30% of total calories. However, not all fats are good for us.

There are four types of fat: monounsaturated, polyunsaturated, saturated, and trans fat. Monounsaturated and polyunsaturated fats are the good fats. I will discuss those two fats in detail in the next chapter. Saturated fat is the unhealthy, bad fat, and trans fat is the artificial, ugly fat.

SATURATED FAT

Medical and government authorities advise that saturated fat is a risk factor for cardiovascular disease and some cancers. Saturated fat is well-known to raise our bad, low-density lipoprotein (LDL) cholesterol levels. What is so bad about LDL cholesterol? It is known to cause plaque deposits in our arteries. If a large piece of plaque breaks loose from one of our arteries, it can clog an artery leading to the heart and cause a heart attack, or clog an artery leading to the brain and cause a stroke. Saturated fat hardens at room temperature. I assume that anything that hardens at room temperature will also harden in my arteries. Saturated fat products are very calorie dense and should only be eaten in moderation.

Some sources of high-calorie, artery-clogging, unhealthy, saturated fat include:

* Whole milk
* Butter
* Lard
* Processed meats (sausage, bologna, salami, etc.)
* Cream
* Fatty meats (like bacon and full-fat hamburger)
* Foods containing hydrogenated oils
* Cheese
* Sour cream
* Ice cream
* Coconut oil
* Palm kernel oil

* Cocoa butter
* Chocolate
* Poultry skin

TRANS FAT

Trans fat is the ugly fat. It is rarely found in nature but can occur in the food production process. Food manufacturers often use trans fat to increase the shelf life of products, and it is also used for deep-frying in many restaurants. Trans fat is associated with coronary heart disease.[17] It is considered by some doctors to be the worst type of fat. Trans fat is known to raise our bad LDL cholesterol while lowering our good, high-density lipoprotein (HDL) cholesterol. The New England Journal of Medicine states that *"the consumption of trans fatty acids results in considerable potential harm but no apparent benefit."* Read product labels. If the label says "partially hydrogenated" anywhere in the ingredients list, chances are good that product contains trans fat. The message is clear: try to avoid processed foods which are loaded full of trans fat.

Some sources of trans fat may include:

* Many fast foods
* Margarine containing partially hydrogenated oils
* Commercial baked goods
* Shortenings
* Some salad dressings
* Cookies
* Many processed breakfast cereals
* Desserts
* Deep-fried foods in some restaurants
* Partially hydrogenated vegetable oils

* Processed foods that say "partially hydrogenated" in the ingredients list

TRANS FAT AND C-REACTIVE PROTEIN (CRP)

C-reactive protein (CRP) is a protein found in the blood. CRP levels rise in response to inflammation in the body. Inflammation is a biological response of vascular tissues to harmful stimuli in the body. A study involving over 700 nurses demonstrated that those in the highest quartile of trans fat consumption had blood levels of CRP that were 73% higher than those in the lowest quartile.[18] In other words, trans-fat consumption causes significant inflammation in the body. Chronic inflammation is a sign of a problem in the body or the makings of one. Research suggests that patients with elevated CRP levels are at increased risk for hypertension, diabetes, and cardiovascular disease.[19][20]

CHOLESTEROL

According to the American Heart Association (AHA), too much cholesterol in the blood can lead to heart disease and stroke, which happen to be America's number one and number three killers. Half of American adults tend to have cholesterol levels that are too high. Most heart disease is caused by a buildup of cholesterol and plaque in the artery walls. It is a well-known fact that saturated fat and trans fat boost the bad LDL cholesterol levels in our blood which can lead to plaque in our arteries. The AHA also recommends limiting foods that are high in cholesterol such as egg yolks. In addition to that, the

AHA recommends losing weight and being physically active to lower cholesterol levels.[21]

Fat-loss strategy #3: Cut down on saturated fat foods. Totally eliminate trans fat from your diet.

PROCESSED FOOD NATION

What are processed foods? In general, processed foods are produced using manufacturing methods to transform raw ingredients from real food into packaged goods using chemical processes. Processed foods are often full of processed sugar, artificial flavors, fillers, artificial sweeteners, saturated fat, trans fat, drugs, high-fructose corn syrup, sodium, chemicals, preservatives, and additives. Needless to say, they don't offer much nutritional value. They are often found in the middle aisles of grocery stores.

What are a few examples of processed foods?

* Candy
* Fried foods
* Processed meat
* Beef jerky
* Potato chips
* Many sugar cereals
* Desserts
* Many canned products
* Many packaged products
* Bottled salad dressings
* Doughnuts

Read the ingredient labels of processed foods, and you might be shocked. Some of chemicals used in processed foods might include the following: nitrates, benzoic acid, sulfur dioxide, butylated hydroxyanisole (BHT), butylated hydroxyanisole (BHA), coal tar, aspartame, propylene glycol, and monosodium glutamate (MSG), just to name a few. Who really knows if these chemicals are safe? For example, propylene glycol is sometimes used as food additive in processed foods and is also a component in newer automotive antifreezes.[22] We are basically being used as guinea pigs when we consume processed foods.

JACK LALANNE AND PROCESSED FOODS

Jack LaLanne was a fitness, exercise, and nutritional expert who passed away in 2011 at the ripe old age of 96. He was extremely fit and healthy right up until the very end. He was known for his numerous books on fitness, his popular TV show, and his amazing physical feats. For example, at age 70, while handcuffed, shackled, and fighting strong winds and currents, he towed 70 rowboats full of guests one mile![23] Not bad at all for a 70-year-old!

Jack blamed processed foods for many health problems. He stressed that chemical food additives and drugs in foods contributed to making people mentally and physically ill. "If man made it, don't eat it" was his philosophy. He stressed the importance of eating good, wholesome foods in proper amounts as close to their natural state as possible. By "natural state," he meant fresh, wholesome food that has been prepared to maintain its full nutritional value as Mother Nature intended.

Does that mean that all processed foods are bad? No, not necessarily. Some processed foods are safe and not bad for our health at all. For example, low-fat milk, oats, frozen 100% fruit juice, canned salmon, canned tuna, frozen vegetables, and some brands of 100% whole-wheat bread. The main thing is to read the product ingredient labels and beware of nasty chemicals like MSG and nitrates. Use your good judgment.

Fat-loss strategy #4: Minimize processed foods as much as possible. Focus on eating wholesome, natural foods in their natural state and in proper amounts.

TOXINS IN OUR ENVIRONMENT

Do you often feel fatigued? Chances are that you may have toxic overload. Let's face it—we live in a very toxic environment. Nasty chemicals are not just in processed foods. Chemicals are in our air, water, homes, offices, cosmetics, creams, lotions, cleaning products, and pharmaceutical drugs, and the list goes on and on. Toxins from the environment can get stored throughout our bodies, especially in the fat cells. How does this hinder our weight-loss efforts? Toxic overload can lead to fatigue and medical problems. Fatigue can lead to food cravings. If you are always feeling fatigued, you are not going to feel like doing much at all, and you certainly are not going to feel like exercising. For example, if you are inhaling cigarette smoke daily, you are filling your body full of toxic chemicals. Chances are very good that you are not going to feel well, and the last thing that you want to do is go to the gym! Keep in mind that too much caffeine and/or alcohol can cause poor sleep and extreme fatigue, which is not what we want when we are trying to lose weight. We can fight back by using water filters, avoiding processed foods, eating organic foods, quitting smoking, and only consuming alcohol and caffeine in moderation. We can also try to be aware of and minimize our exposure to other chemicals in our environment. We can exercise and sweat the toxins out of our bodies. We can also release the toxins from our bodies by losing a lot of fat.

Toxins in food/water environment---->Stored in body fat-------->Toxic overload

Toxic overload----->May lead to medical problems and/or fatigue----->Food cravings----->Weight gain

Lose fat-------->Lose toxins-------->Feel better

SODIUM

Sodium causes water retention, which is not exactly a good thing when you are trying to shed pounds. The maximum recommended daily allowance (RDA) for sodium intake is 2,300 mg. According to the US Department of Agriculture, people with high blood pressure should consume much less than that. Unfortunately, millions of Americans consume far more sodium than they need. According to the Centers for Disease Control (CDC), Americans consume about 3,300 mg of sodium daily on average. Excessive dietary sodium increases blood pressure, which increases the risk for stroke, coronary heart disease, heart failure, and renal disease.[24] That is another reason to avoid processed foods and fast food. They are usually full of sodium. According to the CDC, an astonishing one out of three US adults has high blood pressure. The CDC recommends no more than 1,500 mg of sodium per day if you are in one of the following population groups:[25]

* You are African-American
* You have high blood pressure
* You have diabetes
* You have chronic kidney disease
* You are 51 years of age or older

Talk to your doctor about sodium intake to be sure what is right for you.

Sodium consumed daily

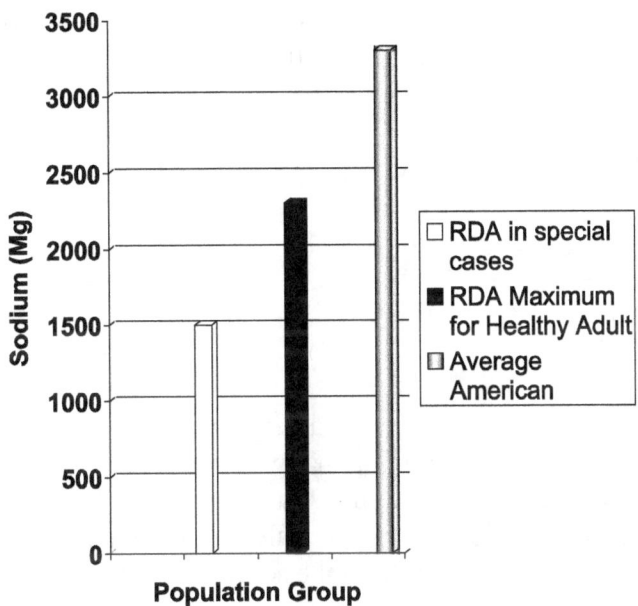

Source: Centers for Disease Control

Fat-loss strategy #5: Minimize sodium in your diet.

I recently examined a typical meal from a popular fast-food chain. The meal was a bacon cheeseburger with regular French fries and a soda. This is typical of what millions of Americans are eating every day:

A TYPICAL FAST-FOOD MEAL

Item	Calories	Sat. Fat (Grams)	Trans Fat (Grams)	Sodium (Mg)
Bacon Cheeseburger	1,090	30	3	2,040
Regular Fries	640	8	10	1,180
Soda (12 oz.)	140	0	0	0
Totals	1,870	38	13	3,220

Notice how this is a very energy-dense meal that is full of everything that we are trying to avoid: calories, saturated fat, trans fat, and sodium, not to mention cholesterol, empty calories, and high-fructose corn syrup from the soda. This is typical of a meal eaten by millions of Americans daily. Is it any wonder that 69% of the population is overweight? Remember that excess sodium can lead to high blood pressure. Just this one fast-food meal exceeds the recommended daily allowance for sodium. Is it any wonder that so many people have high blood pressure? The high-fructose corn syrup in the soda leads to high triglyceride levels and leptin resistance. This meal supplies a whopping 3,220 mg. of sodium, 1,870 calories, and 13 grams of the extremely bad trans fat. Recall that trans fat raises your bad LDL cholesterol and lowers your good HDL cholesterol.

Let's review what we have learned in this chapter. Cut down on empty-calorie, processed carbohydrates and saturated fat products to lose fat.

Totally eliminate trans fat products from your diet. Minimize processed foods in your diet and cut down on salt. So, now we know what to avoid to lose weight. What foods should we be eating for excellent health and weight loss? That is the subject of the next chapter.

CHAPTER 3:

WHAT SHOULD WE BE EATING FOR FAT LOSS AND EXCELLENT HEALTH?

Take care of your body. It's the only place you have to live. —Jom Rohn

In this chapter, I tell you exactly what to eat for energy, fat loss, and excellent health. I also explain a little about spices, phytochemicals, supplements, and the importance of drinking a lot of water. Lastly, I give you some sample diet plans to give you a general idea of what your daily diet might look like to lose fat.

PROTEIN

Protein is the most plentiful substance in the body next to water. It is the major source for building muscles, blood, hair, nails, and internal organs. For energy, the body first burns carbohydrates, then fat, and then protein as a last resort. During digestion, protein is decomposed into simpler units called amino acids. The body requires 22 amino acids to make human protein. All but 8 of those amino acids can be produced in the adult body. Those 8 aminos acids are called "essential amino acids" because they must be supplied in the diet. If just one essential amino acid is missing from the diet, the body is unable to make protein. When a food contains all of the amino acids, it is called a complete protein. Most meats and dairy products are complete proteins, while most fruits and vegetables are incomplete-protein foods. So if you are a vegetarian, you must be very careful to combine various foods to obtain all of the essential amino acids. The National Research Council recommends eating .42 grams of protein for each pound of body weight, so simply multiply your body weight by .42 to get the approximate required daily grams of protein. For example, a 200-pound man needs about 84 grams of protein daily.

FOCUS ON LEAN (LOW-FAT) PROTEIN

Lean protein has little or no saturated fat. We want to focus on egg whites, soy, seafood, fresh-water fish, beans, lean cuts of meat, and skinless poultry. Remember that if you choose to be a vegetarian, you have to carefully combine foods to make sure that you are getting all of the essential amino acids.

TIPS:

* Include a lot of fish in your diet like the Japanese do.

* Trim the excess fat off of your steaks.

* Try to eat lean, organic, grass-fed beef if possible.

* Choose frozen, skinless, chicken tenderloins instead of fatty chicken.

* Choose tuna canned in water instead of tuna canned in oil.

* Buy the lean 90% fat-free hamburger instead of the full fat version.

* Occasionally eat whole eggs but beware of the saturated fat and high cholesterol content.

* Avoid bacon and sausage, which are full of saturated fat and sodium.

* Choose plain soy milk instead of the salty, sugary kind.

* Mackerel, swordfish, tilefish, and shark are known to have high mercury levels, so avoid these.

* Choose wild salmon instead of farmed salmon.

MILK GROUP

We want to focus on low fat or fat free when we choose milk, cheese, yogurt, and other milk products.

TIPS:

* Whole milk fattens baby cows and will fatten you up very quickly, so avoid it.

* Choose sugar-free, plain yogurt instead of sweetened yogurt (you can add fruit at home to sweeten).

COMPLEX CARBOHYDRATES

Complex carbohydrates are the healthy (good) carbs. They are high-fiber foods that are full of vitamins and minerals, are slow to digest, and they very slowly release glucose (energy) throughout the day. Complex carbs stabilize your blood sugar and help you to feel satisfied longer after a meal. Unlike processed carbs that have very few nutrients, complex carbs are packed full nutrients that our bodies need for good health. Here are some examples of complex carbs:

* Oatmeal
* Soy milk
* Wild rice
* Navy beans
* Vegetables
* Pinto beans
* Kidney beans
* Soybcans
* Multi-grain bread
* Buckwheat bread
* Oat bran bread
* Whole-grain rice
* Whole barley
* Oat bran cereal
* Whole-grain pasta
* Lentils

GRAINS TIPS:

* Choose whole-grain bread instead of white bread.

* Choose whole-grain pasta instead of white, processed pasta.

* Choose oatmeal instead of sugary breakfast cereal (add a touch of honey or fruit to oats for flavor).

* Try to avoid boiling your vegetables because that leaches out the nutrients.

EAT ALL FRUITS

We want to focus on eating a big variety of fruits and vegetables in a big variety of colors. These are water-dense foods, and water has zero calories. These fill you up and are packed full of fiber, vitamins, minerals, and other nutrients that our bodies need for good health.

TIPS:

* Choose fresh, frozen, or dried fruits and vegetables instead of the sugary, canned ones if possible.

* Fruit and vegetable juices are OK as long as they are not loaded with high-fructose corn syrup, added artificial sweeteners, salt, and/or processed sugar. Look for product labels that say 100% juice.

PHYTOCHEMICALS

Did you know that plants contain naturally occurring chemical compounds called phytochemicals? To date, scientists estimate that there may be as many as 10,000 different phytochemicals that have the potential to affect diseases such as cancer. Many phytochemicals are currently being tested as potential treatments for a variety of diseases. We generally only hear about vitamins like A, B, C, D, E, and K, and minerals, but fruits, vegetables, grains, beans, and other plants are full of these phytochemicals, most of which have not even been identified yet. When you eat an orange, you are getting a dose of vitamin C, and you are also getting a dose of phytochemicals. Simply popping a vitamin C pill does not give you all of these nutrients. Some of the well-known phytochemicals are lycopene found in tomatoes, isoflavones found in soy, and flavonoids in fruits. A single carrot may contain over 100 phytochemicals. Eat a big variety of fruits, vegetables, beans, and grains to get all of these nutrients.

Phytochemicals may be destroyed or removed by modern processing techniques. That's another reason to avoid processed foods when possible. White bread and white pasta are examples of foods that have been processed and stripped of any nutritional value. That's why it is always best to eat 100% whole-wheat products.

The greatest wealth is health. —Virgil

HEALTHY FATS

Fat is very high in calories. For example, just a tablespoon of olive oil contains about 120 calories, but remember that we need some fat in the diet for good health. The American Heart Association recommends that no more than 25–35% of our daily calories should come from fat and that we should mostly eat the healthy monounsaturated and polyunsaturated fats:

(1) MONOUNSATURATED FAT

Monounsaturated fat is usually liquid at room temperature. It has been shown to reduce the harmful, low-density, lipoprotein (LDL) cholesterol in our bodies and possibly cause an increase in the good, high-density lipoprotein (HDL) cholesterol, which helps to lower your risk of heart disease and stroke. Monounsaturated fats are typically high in vitamin E, an antioxidant that most people need more of. It is found in avocados, olives, oatmeal, whole-grain wheat, popcorn, many nuts and seeds, many fish, peanut butter, and olive, canola, sunflower, safflower, soybean, and peanut oils.

(2) POLYUNSATURATED FAT

Polyunsaturated fat is also liquid at room temperature. Omega-3 and Omega-6 fatty acids are two types of polyunsaturated fat. Omega-3 fatty acid is found in fish and has been shown to lower the risk of heart attacks.[26] Omega-6 fatty acid is found in sunflower seeds and safflower oil and may reduce the risk of cardiovascular disease. Some other good sources of polyunsaturated fat include walnuts, peanuts, flax oil, soybean and corn oils.

TIPS:

* Cook with canola oil instead of lard or butter.

* Flavor your salads with a touch of olive oil instead of sugary dressings that often have trans fat.

* Choose nuts and seeds with no added salt instead of the salty options.

* Go easy on the fats because they are very high in calories (just one tablespoon of oil might have 120 calories).

SPICES

Just because we are eating healthy foods, that does not mean that our food has to be bland. Spices are packed full of healthy nutrients, and the calories are practically zero.

RECOMMENDED SPICES:

Garlic, chili powder, cloves, oregano, basil, black pepper, red pepper, tarragon, *cayenne pepper, lemon pepper, paprika, curry powder, ginger, nutmeg, onion powder, sweet basil, thyme, mustard, rosemary, lime, savory, onion, parsley, cinnamon, sage, bay leaves, sea salt (in moderation)**, and chives.

    *Note 1: Some people swear by cayenne pepper for weight loss because it supposedly speeds up your metabolism.
    **Note 2: Excess salt is not recommended.

I tried every diet in the book. I tried some that weren't in the book. I tried eating the book. It tasted better than most of the diets. —Dolly Parton

SPICE THINGS UP! GO FOR THE FLAVOR!

You do not have to eat sugary, salty junk food to get a lot of flavor. Spices are packed full of nutrients. Use your imagination and add spices to a lot of your foods. Here are some examples:

* Add cinnamon to plain yogurt or oatmeal.
* Add salsa to scrambled eggs.
* Add vanilla to skim milk.
* Add a lemon to plain water.
* Add lemon pepper to salad.
* Add nutmeg to peaches.
* Add chili to sandwiches.
* Add curry to low-salt sauces.
* Add red pepper to lean chicken.
* Add black pepper to lean steaks.
* Replace sugar with cinnamon, nutmeg, or vanilla spice.

DRINK A LOT OF WATER

The human body is made of 55–75% water. Just a small water deficiency can cause tiredness, affect athletic ability, and dull critical-thinking abilities. Most people don't drink nearly enough water. Water will energize you, fill you up when you are hungry, and also give you beautiful skin. Best of all, water has zero calories.

Some symptoms of mild dehydration include headaches, little or no urination, dizziness, irritability, dry skin, muscle weakness, grogginess, constipation, dry mouth, thirst or hunger, lack of sweating, and sometimes insomnia. If you are suffering from any of these symptoms, you may not be drinking enough water.

How much water should you drink daily? Use the 8 x 8 rule. Drink eight or more eight-ounce glasses of filtered water daily. If you are trying to lose weight, it might be a great idea to drink even more because water fills you up quenches any hunger pangs. Of course, you also want to eat a lot of water-dense foods like fruits and vegetables instead of calorie-dense foods like saturated fat products.

TIP: Drink filtered water instead of regular tap water or sugary, high-calorie colas and other high-calorie beverages.

Fat-loss strategy #6: Drink several glasses of filtered water every day. Replace sugary colas and other high-calorie drinks with filtered water. Water will fill you up when you feel hungry and has zero calories.

SUPPLEMENTS FOR HEALTH

* Multivitamins/minerals are beneficial. Many people are deficient in some vitamin or mineral and don't even realize it. That deficiency might lead to several health problems. Think of taking a vitamin/mineral supplement as an insurance policy against any deficiencies. But realize that you are not getting the beneficial phytochemicals found in plants when you simply pop an artificial pill.

* L-carnitine is an amino acid that has been shown to reduce triglycerides. Remember that high triglycerides in the blood cause leptin resistance. In a three-month study of diabetes patients by researchers Mariano Malaguarnera, Marco Vacante, et al., published in *The American Journal of Clinical Nutrition,* 81 patients were randomly divided into two groups.[27] One group was given two grams of L-carnitine daily, and the other group was given a placebo. After three months, the L-carnitine group showed significant decreases in triglycerides and bad LDL cholesterol. Furthermore, the L-carnitine group showed a significant increase in the good HDL cholesterol.

* Flax oil is a good source of the omega-3 fatty acids that have been shown to reduce triglycerides.

* Green tea has many health benefits and is full of antioxidants. At least one study discovered that green tea extract significantly helps with weight loss.[28] Green tea extract is found in some weight-loss products. Recall that the Japanese drink a lot of green tea instead of soda. Just remember that green tea has caffeine, so moderation is the key.

THE MIRACLE OF L-ARGININE AND NITRIC OXIDE

Dr. Louis Ignarro and colleagues were awarded the Nobel Prize in Medicine in 1998 for the discovery of the importance of nitric oxide (NO) to the cardiovascular system. NO is a tiny molecule that is specifically produced by the body to keep arteries free of plaque and to maintain normal blood pressure. L-arginine is an essential amino acid that is converted by the body into NO. You can buy L-arginine supplements at any health-food store. Dr. Ignarro recommends combining L-arginine with another amino acid called L-citrulline for optimal results.

Well, the news for L-arginine just keeps getting better and better. In a 2006 study by Pietro Lucotti, Emanuela Setola, et al. that was published by the American Physiology Society, 33 obese type 2 diabetic patients were placed on a hypocaloric diet and an exercise program.[29] The patients were randomly divided into two groups. The first group received 8.3 grams/day of L-arginine and the second group received a placebo. The experiment lasted for 21 days. Results: both groups lost significant and similar amounts of weight. However, in the L-arginine group, fat loss accounted for 100% of the total weight loss. In the placebo group, muscle loss accounted for 43% of the total weight loss and fat loss accounted for only 57%. In other words, L-arginine helps spare muscle while you lose weight. That's a huge finding! Weight training also helps you to spare muscle as you lose weight. Furthermore, the L-arginine group lost three times as much size around the waist as the placebo group. As if that is not exciting enough, blood pressure significantly declined in the L-arginine group, while there was virtually no change in the placebo group.

It's a well-known fact that L-arginine causes the pituitary gland to secrete growth hormone (GH). One of the many functions of GH is to maintain or increase muscle mass in our bodies. GH is also known to reduce body fat. That explains why the obese patients on L-arginine were able to maintain their muscle while losing only fat. Secretion of GH naturally declines as we age. Some people actually get injected with GH as a "fountain of youth," but more research needs to be done.

As a side note, I decided to put L-arginine to the test myself. I have been taking six grams/day for several months. Nothing in my routine has changed other than me taking L-arginine. I have noticed that my body fat is getting extremely low and that my running times have significantly improved. It makes sense that my running times would improve because L-arginine improves circulation by increasing NO production. It also makes sense that I am getting extremely lean because L-arginine causes the secretion of GH. I have yet to try combining L-arginine with L-citrulline for a synergetic effect like Dr. Ignarro recommends, but I plan to do so in the future. It's worth taking L-arginine just for the beneficial cardiovascular effects like keeping your arteries free of plaque and lowering blood pressure. The fat-loss effects are icing on the cake.

L-arginine--->Increases nitric oxide--->Improves cardiovascular health

L-arginine--->Increases growth hormone--->Spares muscle as you lose fat

DIET EXAMPLES FOR FAT LOSS

(DIET EXAMPLE #1):

BREAKFAST   (ESTIMATED CALORIES)

3 egg whites (cooked with dab of canola oil) (68)
1 bowl of oatmeal (with blueberries) (205)
Glass of 100% orange juice (111)

MID-MORNING SNACKS

1 Orange (62)
Several glasses of filtered water (0)

LUNCH

Salad with raw spinach, broccoli, carrots,
mushrooms, spices, olive oil (172)
Small handful of walnuts on salad (60)
Large glass of filtered water with lemon slice (0)

AFTERNOON SNACKS

1 small handful of sunflower seeds (150)
Several glasses of filtered water (0)

DINNER

Chicken tenderloins cooked in dab of canola oil with
spices (160)
1 serving of brown rice with spices (130)
1 serving of broccoli with spices (24)
1 cup of skim milk (86)

TOTAL CALORIES   (1,228)

(DIET EXAMPLE #2)

BREAKFAST   (ESTIMATED CALORIES)

1 bowl of plain yogurt (add cinnamon spice) (139)
1 small handful of unsalted almonds (190)
1 banana (105)
1 slice of 100% whole-wheat toast (add honey) (110)
1 cup of hot green tea (0)

MID-MORNING SNACKS

1 apple (81)
Rice cake (salt-free) (35)
Several glasses of filtered water (0)

LUNCH

Turkey (4 ounces) sandwich with 100% whole-wheat
bread and mustard (240)
1 serving of kidney beans (109)
Iced tea with a lemon slice (0)

AFTERNOON SNACKS

1/2 cup of blueberries (41)
Several glasses of filtered water (0)

DINNER

Raw spinach, cucumbers, mushrooms, parsley, olive
oil and spices (156)
Grilled salmon (4 ounces) with spices (246)
1 cup of skim milk (86)

TOTAL CALORIES   (1,538)

We want to focus on eating lean protein, low-fat dairy, fruits, complex carbs, and healthy fats, and drinking a lot of water.

A diet is the penalty we pay for exceeding the feed limit. —Unknown

In order to help you successfully count calories, I have listed the calorie content of common healthy foods that you should be eating for weight loss. There are also many free websites that tell you the amount of calories in many common foods. One such website is **caloriecount.about.com**.

BAKERY AND GRAINS (estimated calories)

Bread 100% whole-wheat (56)
Oatmeal 1/2 cup (150)
Pasta 100% whole-wheat 1 cup (174)
Pita 100% whole-wheat (140)
Popcorn plain 1 cup (54)
Rice brown 3/4 cup (130)
Rice cakes salt free 1 (35)
Rice white 3/4 cup (181)
Rice wild 1 cup (164)
Roll 100% whole wheat (90)

DAIRY AND EGGS (estimated calories)

Cheese cheddar (reduced-fat) 28 grams (80)
Cheese Swiss (reduced-fat) 21 grams (70)
Cottage cheese (low-fat) 1/2 cup (100)
Egg whole (in moderation) (79)

Egg white 1 egg (16)
Kefir plain (low-fat) 1 cup (120)
Milk skim 1 cup (86)
Yogurt (low-fat) 1 cup (144)
Yogurt plain 1 cup (139)

FATS AND OILS (estimated calories)

Canola oil 1 tbsp (120)
Olive oil 1 tbsp (120)
Safflower oil 1 tbsp (120)
Smart Balance® spread 1 tbsp (80)

FRUITS AND FRUIT JUICES (estimated calories)

Apple (81)
Apple juice 100% 1 cup (116)
Apricot (51)
Avocado 1/2 (162)
Banana (105)
Blackberries 1/2 cup (37)
Blueberries 1/2 cup (41)
Cantaloupe 1/2 (94)
Cherries 1/2 cup (52)
Grapefruit 1/2 (38)
Grapefruit juice 100% 1 cup (96)
Grapes 1/2 cup (29)
Grape juice 100% 1 cup (155)
Honeydew melon 1/10 (50)
Orange (62)
Orange juice 100% 1 cup (111)
Peach (37)
Pear (98)

Plum (36)
Raisins 14 grams (42)
Raspberries 1/2 cup (30)
Strawberries 1/2 cup (23)

MEATS (estimated calories)

Ground beef (93% lean) 1/4 pound (203)
Round steak lean 1/4 pound (216)

NUTS AND SEEDS (estimated calories)

Almonds 1/4 cup (212)
Cashews 1/4 cup (196)
Peanuts 1/4 cup (209)
Peanut butter plain 1 tbsp (86)
Pecans 1/4 cup (185)
Pistachios shelled 1/4 cup (184)
Pumpkin seeds 1/4 cup (193)
Sunflower seeds 1/4 cup (203)
Walnuts 1/4 cup (162)

POULTRY (estimated calories)

Chicken light meat w/o skin 1/4 pound (90)
Turkey lean light meat 52 grams (60)

SALAD DRESSINGS AND SAUCES (estimated calories)

Italian (fat-free) dressing (20)
Catsup 1 tbsp (16)

Horseradish 1 tbsp (6)
Margarine (w/zero trans fat) 1 tbsp (80)
Mayonnaise (reduced fat) 1 tbsp (25)
Mustard 1 tbsp (15)
Ranch dressing (fat-free) (48)
Salsa 1 tbsp (36)
Soy 1 tbsp (11)
Tomato paste 1/2 cup (107)

SEAFOOD (estimated calories)

Catfish 1/4 pound (117)
Cod 1/4 pound (88)
Crab 1/4 pound (105)
Halibut 1/4 pound (113)
Herring 1/4 pound (200)
Lobster 1/4 pound (103)
Salmon 1/4 pound (246)
Scallops 1/4 pound (91)
Shrimp 1/4 pound (103)
Snapper 1/4 pound (105)
Trout 1/4 pound (221)
Tuna (5 ounces) canned in water (50)

VEGETABLES AND VEGETABLE JUICES (estimated calories)

Artichoke medium (65)
Asparagus 1/2 cup (15)
Black eye peas cooked 1/2 cup (89)
Broccoli 1/2 cup (12)
Brussels sprouts 1/2 cup (19)
Carrots 1/2 cup (24)
Carrot juice 100% 1 cup (96)

Cauliflower 1/2 cup (12)
Celery 1/2 cup (9)
Corn 1/2 cup (66)
Cucumber 1/2 cup (7)
Eggplant 1/2 cup (11)
Green beans 1/2 cup (17)
Kidney beans cooked 1/2 cup (109)
Lentils cooked 1/2 cup (106)
Lettuce romaine 1/2 cup (4)
Lima beans cooked 1/2 cup (104)
Mushrooms 1/2 cup (9)
Navy beans cooked 1/2 cup (112)
Okra 1/2 cup (19)
Onions 1/2 cup (27)
Parsley 1/2 cup (13)
Peas green 1/2 cup (59)
Peppers sweet 1/2 cup (12)
Pickles dill 1 large (11)
Pinto beans cooked 1/2 cup (122)
Potato (w/skin) 1 large (110)
Radish quantity 10 (10)
Soybeans cooked 1/2 cup (117)
Spinach 1 cup (7)
Sweet potato 1 (136)
Tomato 1 (24)
Tomato juice 100% 1 cup (46)
Watercress 1 cup (7)
Yams 1/2 cup (105)

Notice that most fruits and vegetables are extremely low in calories. For example, one full cup of raw spinach has only 7 calories, and half a cup of broccoli on has 15 calories. Eating and digesting these healthy foods probably uses up more than the calorie intake. So spinach and broccoli are actually negative-calorie foods! Add some more veggies and spices along with a touch of olive oil to the spinach and broccoli, and you have a great-tasting, filling, low-calorie meal with probably less than 175 calories. Compare that with a cheeseburger at the local fast-food joint that might easily have over 700 calories.

KEY POINT: *When forced to eat out, go for the salads. Just beware of the salad dressings, cheese, bacon bits, and croutons, which might be high in calories, saturated fat, trans fat, and sodium.*

TIP:

* If you like margarine, look for a spread that has zero trans fat and is low in saturated fat. Some spreads contain the healthy olive and/or canola oils.

WHAT ARE SOME LOW-CALORIE SNACKS TO FILL YOU UP?

It seems that a lot of dieters know that they should be cutting calories to lose weight, but they give in to their hunger cravings. The trick is to find low-calorie snacks that fill you up and satisfy those cravings. These snacks are great to handle any cravings and fill you up:

* Plain popcorn
* Plain yogurt
* All fruits and vegetables
* Rice cakes

* Fresh veggies with salsa
* Apple slices with cinnamon
* Fruit smoothie
* Frozen fruit (grapes or blueberries for example)
* Half a can of red kidney beans with salsa
* Water with a lemon slice

In summary, we want to eat a big variety of healthy foods to ensure that we get all of the necessary vitamins, minerals, protein, carbs, and healthy fats. We want to focus on eating lean protein, fruits, low-fat dairy, complex carbs, and healthy fats, and drinking a lot of water. In the next chapter, I explain our metabolisms and help you determine how many calories to actually cut from your daily diet to safely lose weight.

CHAPTER 4:

OUR METABOLISMS AND COUNTING CALORIES

One may walk over the highest mountain one step at a time. —John Wanamaker

In chapter 1, I explained how we must cut calories to lose weight. In this chapter, I explain our metabolisms and help you determine how many calories that you should actually cut from your daily diet to safely lose weight. As a general rule, most experts agree that losing two pounds of fat per week is a reasonable and safe goal. Remember one pound of fat equals 3,500 calories, and two pounds of fat equals 7,000 calories. So, to lose two pounds of fat per week, we need to create a daily calorie deficit of 1,000 calories, which equals a deficit of 7,000 calories/week.

If you have been exercising and stuck at the same bodyweight for years, that means that your calorie consumption equals your calorie expenditure. If your goal is to lose weight, you either need to exercise more and/or cut your calories. By far, the easiest way to shed fat is to simply cut calories from your daily diet. It's a lot easier to just avoid that 1,000-calorie snack than it is to go out and run 10 miles. The good news is that if you simply eliminate the processed, empty-calorie carbs from your diet, cut down on processed foods, cut down on the high-calorie, saturated-fat foods, and eliminate trans fat from your diet, you will likely create a calorie deficit and begin to lose weight.

HOW WEIGHT CAN GRADUALLY SNEAK UP ON US

If we regularly consume an average of just 150 extra calories per day, that might not seem like much. But that adds up to about 7.8 pounds of fat in just six months. That amounts to 15.6 pounds of fat in just one year. Fat is nothing but stored energy (calories). Over two years, we will have gained 31 pounds of fat just from an average of 150 excess calories per day. You might think nothing of regularly adding that extra ranch dressing to your salad, adding extra mayonnaise to your daily sandwich, having bacon for breakfast, or drinking that extra soda daily, but those high-density calories really add up over time.

Happily, we can reverse this process by eliminating the high-density foods and replacing them with low-density foods. Instead of a 150-calorie surplus every day, we can create a 150-calorie deficit every day. Better yet, we can really watch our diets and exercise, and create a 500-calorie deficit or even a 1,000-calorie daily deficit to really speed up the process of losing fat.

Some people are very confused about how low they should actually drop their calorie consumption to safely lose weight. As a general rule of thumb, you never want to drop your daily calories below 1,200 because your body will think that you are starving and go into "famine mode." Your metabolism will slow down. Also, we need a certain amount of nutrients in our daily diet for good health. We might develop nutritional deficiencies if we drop our daily calories too low. What exactly do I mean by metabolism or basal metabolic rate?

BASAL METABOLIC RATE (BMR)

Basal metabolic rate (BMR) is the amount of daily energy (calories) expended by humans at rest. Our bodies and organs are constantly burning calories just to function. Blood circulation, breathing, digestion, and organ function all burn calories. As a matter of fact, basal metabolism burns about 80% of our daily calories![30] Our organs burn 70%, and digestion burns 10%. The remaining 20% of our calories are burned by daily activities. So, say that we are eating 2,400 calories/day and maintaining our bodyweight. Our metabolism burns up an amazing 1,920 calories/day! Exercise from daily activities burns up the remaining 480 calories. Of course, if we don't get any exercise at all, those excess 480 calories are stored as fat.

KEY POINT: *Our basal metabolism is usually by far the largest component of our daily calorie expenditure (about 80%).*

HOW DO WE SPEED UP OUR METABOLISMS?

* An effective way to boost our metabolisms is with

weight training. Muscle burns more calories than fat, and the more muscle that we build, the more calories that we burn at rest maintaining that muscle. Men have faster metabolisms than women because men have more muscle than women.[31] As we age, our metabolisms slow down, mostly because we lose muscle. But there is no reason that we have to lose muscle if we train with weights.

* Don't starve yourself. Dropping your calories to below 1,200 per day will signal to your body that you are in a famine, and your metabolism will slow down.

* Aerobic exercise, especially interval training, has the added benefit of speeding up your metabolism for four to eight hours after you exercise. What is interval training? It is bursts of high-intensity moves. For example, walk or run on the incline treadmill at a very fast pace for maybe one minute. Slow down the pace and walk slowly for a minute. Then repeat the process several times. I explain interval training in detail in chapter 6.

* Exercise twice per day. That's not as daunting as it sounds. For example, you could do a quick 15-minute workout in the morning before work and then walk for 30 minutes during your lunch break. That speeds up your metabolism twice per day.

* Have four to five very small meals instead of one or two large meals. Digesting those four to five small meals keeps your metabolism working hard and running in high gear all day long.

HOW FAR SHOULD WE DROP OUR DAILY CALORIES TO LOSE FAT?

We have established that we need to cut our calorie intake to lose weight. The question is, how far should we actually drop our daily calorie intake to safely lose fat?

There are two ways that we can get a rough idea of how low to drop our daily calorie consumption:

(1) Trial and error

You can experiment and watch your results. If you are not seeing results, your calorie consumption is too high, or you are not getting enough exercise. If you are losing more than two to three pounds per week, you are probably losing muscle along with the fat unless you are extremely obese. So, you can adjust your calories and exercise accordingly until you see the results that you want.

(2) Rule of thumb

Multiply your weight by 11 to figure out how many calories to eat to MAINTAIN your weight. For example, if you weigh 200 pounds, multiply 200 x 11 = 2200 calories. That's assuming no exercise. Of course, if you want to lose weight, drop your calories way below that maintenance level and exercise. For weight loss:

Women who weigh less than 250 pounds should aim for 1,200 calories per day.
Women who weigh 250–300 pounds should aim for 1,600 calories per day.
Women who weigh more than 300 pounds should aim for 1,800 calories per day.

Men who weigh less than 250 pounds should aim for 1,400 calories per day.
Men who weigh 250–300 pounds should aim for 1,600 calories per day.
Men who weigh more than 300 pounds should aim for 1,800 calories per day.

Recall that I gave an example of a typical fast-food meal in chapter 2. Just that one meal contained 1,870 calories. Clearly, if losing weight is your goal, you will need to avoid fast-food restaurants. I understand that you might be forced to eat out often. In that case, go for the salads. Just go easy on the cheese, dressings, bacon bits, and croutons.

SPINNING YOUR WHEELS

You might be working out every day, exercising like crazy, and eating the healthiest diet in the world, but if you are eating a ton of calories, you are just spinning your wheels. You will not lose any weight at all if your calorie consumption equals or exceeds your calorie expenditure. This is so obvious that most dieters overlook it. People think that just because they are exercising and eating healthfully, they must lose weight, but the scale never budges.

Even healthy food has calories. I can't stress to you enough that you have got to cut your calories to shed the fat.

KEY POINT: *If you have been exercising and have been stuck at the same weight for months or even years, it means that your daily calorie consumption equals your daily calorie expenditure. Try to cut your current calorie intake by 500–1,000 calories per day to lose one to two pounds per week, but never go below 1,200 calories/day.*

CASE STUDY

Mary weighed 180 pounds and was very frustrated because she could not lose weight, no matter what she tried. She spent countless hours on the stair machine at the gym and performed other exercises. She tried to eat healthy foods as much as possible. However, the scale never budged. She was ready to give up.

She finally asked me what she was doing wrong. I explained to her that even healthy food has calories, and she needed to cut calories to shed the fat. No doubt, she was burning a lot of calories at the gym, but she was also eating 2,000 or more calories/day. I advised her to keep exercising and cut her calories down to 1,200/day, and she began losing fat very quickly.

I saw her again several months later, and she looked amazing. She was at least 30 pounds lighter and had a big grin on her face.

__Fat-loss strategy #7: Women who weigh less than 250 pounds should aim for 1,200 calories/day. Men who weigh less than 250 pounds should aim for 1,400 calories/day. Both men and women who weigh 250–300 pounds should aim for 1,600 calories/day. Both men and women who weigh over 300 pounds should aim for 1,800 calories/day.__

CHAPTER 5:

EXERCISE FOR FAT LOSS

*Exercise is good for your mind, body, and soul. —
Susie Michelle Cortright*

Exercise is important for fat loss. Many people have no energy or motivation to exercise. In this chapter, I explain why some people have no energy and how to get energized. I try to get you motivated to exercise by explaining the benefits of exercise and the importance of choosing a good exercise partner and a fitness program that you enjoy. Many people get stuck in a plateau where progress grinds to a halt. I tell you how to break through that plateau.

I realize that there are many people out there with serious health issues, so always get permission from your doctor before beginning any exercise routine.

But I have no energy to exercise!! What should I do?

I can understand that. In chapter 2, I wrote about the importance of eliminating toxins from your environment to experience more energy and better health. Also, consider that if you are 50 pounds overweight, that is like carrying around a 50-pound bag of cement around with you 24 hours per day. Anybody would be exhausted from carrying around a 50-pound bag of cement. If you currently have a horrible diet full of greasy fast food, colas, salt, white sugar, and processed food, then of course you are to feel lousy and not have much energy. If you smoke cigarettes, you must quit. Your energy and health will drastically improve.

The good news is that once you start changing your diet and drinking a lot of filtered water, you will begin to experience more energy. Once you start exercising and sweating out all of those toxins from your body, you will begin to feel so much better and probably sleep better. Once that fat starts melting off, you will be hauling less weight around. Can you imagine how much more energy you will have once you are not carrying around that 50-pound bag of cement? You will feel light as a feather!

What else might be causing your lack of energy?

CAFFEINE AND ADRENAL EXHAUSTION

You don't have to explain your caffeine addiction to me. I was a caffeine addict for years. I got to the point where I was easily drinking a pot per day of coffee. I was always stressed out and not sleeping well. Large amounts of caffeine may stay in the body for up to 24 hours. I decided to quit cold turkey. Of course, I experienced withdrawal symptoms. I had headaches for several days because caffeine causes blood vessels to constrict, especially in the brain. The headaches were caused by the blood vessels in my brain slowly returning back to normal. In hindsight, I could have avoided the headaches by gradually cutting the caffeine instead of quitting cold turkey. I replaced the coffee with a drink that tastes like coffee but without the caffeine. Now that I quit, I feel like a new person, and I am definitely sleeping better. Just one cup of coffee may not affect you much, but many people drink much more than that, and caffeine is also found in colas, chocolate, energy drinks, etc. Over time, that daily caffeine exhausts our adrenal glands.

Our adrenal glands secrete cortisol, adrenalin, androgens (like DHEA), and other hormones. Caffeine causes the adrenal glands to secrete large amounts of adrenalin and cortisol, which are stress hormones. That's why we feel the "pickup" in the mornings from that cup of coffee. Caffeine is a drug, and over time some people may develop a tolerance to it similar to what happens with other drugs. Eventually, people need more and more caffeine to get the same pickup and the adrenals become exhausted from cranking out those stress hormones every day. As adrenal function declines, a person becomes more and more chronically tired. Large amounts of caffeine slowly wear out the adrenal glands. It becomes a vicious cycle. As the stress response dissipates during the day, people may feel more tired and hungry. They reach for a "sugar fix" or more caffeine to get another quick pickup.

Poor sleep---------->Drink caffeine to wakeup--------- --->Cortisol/adrenalin--->Stressed out--->Poor sleep

Caffeine--->Stress hormones daily--->Adrenal exhaustion----->Chronically tired

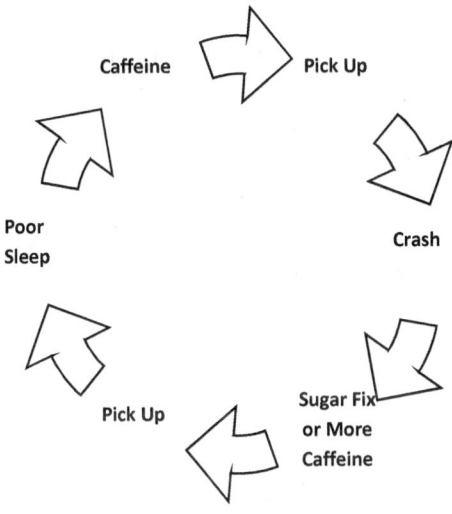

Caffeine is found in many weight-loss supplements, and it probably does temporarily speed up your metabolism. However, moderation is the key. Keep in mind that if you are currently drinking way too much caffeine, it might be interfering with your mood, adrenals, and sleep quality, which could leave you feeling drained and low on energy every day. Being chronically exhausted means no energy for exercise or anything else. If you would like to know more about the effects of caffeine, I highly recommend the book *Caffeine Blues* by Stephen Cherniske, MS.

BENEFITS OF EXERCISE FOR YOU

Not only is exercise highly recommended for

any successful weight-loss program, but exercise is the fountain of youth. As we age, our bodies lose muscle and bone density, and gain fat. Our metabolisms slow down, and we lose heart and lung power. Exercise directly counteracts all of those signs of aging. Exercise builds muscle, strengthens bones, burns fat, strengthens our heart and lungs, and speeds up our metabolism for several hours after exercising. That means that we are burning extra calories for several hours after we work out. If you really want to look your best, and tone and shape your body, exercise is a must.

BETTER SLEEP

Many people suffer from insomnia. As a matter of fact, one poll by the National Sleep Foundation showed that 58% of adults in the U.S. experience insomnia at least a few nights per week. The good news is that exercise can help you fall asleep faster and sleep better. Cutting down on salt and caffeine might help too. Many people are surprised to learn that salt is a stimulant just like caffeine. Too much salt during the day can keep you awake at night.

Sleep apnea is a sleep disorder characterized by abnormal breathing during sleep. Obstructive sleep apnea (OSA) is the most common type of sleep-disordered breathing. The risk of OSA increases with age, smoking, and bodyweight. Individuals with low muscle tone and soft tissue around the airway (from obesity) are at high risk for OSA. Symptoms include restless sleep, snoring, and feeling tired during the day.

YOUR SKIN WILL LOOK GREAT

Once you start drinking a lot of water and replacing the junk food in your diet with foods like salmon, cantaloupe, and carrots, your skin will start to look much healthier. Salt from fast food and processed junk dehydrates our bodies, including the skin.

EXERCISE DOES BECOME EASIER

I realize that exercise is very difficult at first, especially if you have not exercised in a while, but the good news is that it becomes much easier as you gradually get into shape. I used to hate running, but once I saw the results and got into shape, I really began to enjoy running. It became much easier. It's so easy to get addicted to the endorphins. But unlike some other addictions, exercise is good for us. If you want to look and feel 10 years younger, regular exercise will help you do that.

Here are just a few more benefits of exercise:

* Do you need an emotional lift? Exercise improves mood.

* Do you need to blow off some steam after a stressful day? Exercise will let you do that.

* Are you often lethargic and low on energy?

Exercise will boost your energy.

* Do you want to boost your healthy HDL cholesterol and lower your bad LDL cholesterol? Exercise will do that.

* Do you often have trouble falling or staying asleep? Exercise promotes better sleep.

* Do you have a slow metabolism? Exercise temporarily speeds up your metabolism.

KEY POINT: *People who lose weight and keep it off are people who exercise regularly. Diet without exercise is not good because you end up losing a lot of muscle along with the fat. There's no reason for the body to maintain muscle while dieting if you are not exercising.*

WALKING

Walking is probably the best option to start with for most people who are trying to lose weight. It's easy on the joints and easy to stick with the exercise program. You can start with a small distance of, say, half a mile to one mile per day. Do that for at least three to four days per week and gradually work your way up to three to four miles for at least five days per week. Walk everywhere. Walk to the store or work if possible. Walk around the park. Walk the dog. Walk around the track, at the beach, or on the treadmill. Park farther away from your destinations and walk. If you are really out of shape, you may want to start with the beginner routine (below) and gradually increase your time and distance as you lose fat and get into shape.

Beginner routine:

Walk for 30 minutes, 4–5 days/week.

Intermediate routine:

Walk for 45 minutes, 5 days/week.

Advanced routine:

Walk/run for 1 hour, 5–6 days/week.

Even if you are on the right track, you'll get run over if you just sit there. —Will Rogers

SEASONAL AFFECTIVE DISORDER (SAD)

SAD is a mood disorder in which people with normal mental health throughout most of the year experience depressive symptoms during the winter months due to lack of sunlight. Some experts say that SAD may affect as many as 10–20% of Americans. That's a lot of people! Some of the effects of SAD may include the following symptoms:

* Lack of energy
* Difficulty waking
* Difficulty concentrating
* Depression
* Withdrawal from friends and family
* **Craving for refined carbohydrates**

* **Overeating**
* **Weight gain**

Lack of sunlight------>Depression------>Craving for refined carbs------>Overeating------>Weight gain

Furthermore, many people who don't get enough sunlight are deficient in vitamin D, which is manufactured by the body when exposed to sunlight. Walking outdoors is a great way to burn fat, combat SAD, and boost your vitamin D levels all at the same time. As little as 15 minutes outdoors in the sunlight is enough to ease the symptoms of SAD. Too much of a good thing can cause melanoma, so moderate exposure to sunlight is the key.

AEROBIC AND ANAEROBIC EXERCISE

Aerobic exercise is any type of exercise that gets the heart pumping for a long period, such as running, fast walking, biking, swimming, or aerobic classes. It really works the heart and lungs, and burns a lot of calories.

Anaerobic exercise does not necessarily get the heart rate up for an extended period. It is used to tone the body, build muscle in all of the right places, and strengthen the bones. Increased muscle speeds up the metabolism and shapes the body. Some examples of anaerobic exercise are push-ups, sit-ups, pull-ups, Pilates, and weight training.

A key benefit of anaerobic training is that it helps you to preserve muscle while losing weight on a low-calorie diet. If you simply diet without exercising, the body tends to lose a lot of muscle along with the fat. Losing muscle is not a good thing. Preserve muscle with exercise.

Recall that I wrote about L-arginine helping to preserve muscle mass while on a low-calorie diet. The dieters who took L-arginine lost 100% fat, while the placebo group lost 47% muscle and 53% fat. Also, the L-arginine dieters lost three times as much size around the waist as the placebo group. So you may want to add an L-arginine supplement to your diet as well as some form of anaerobic training to your routine.

For best results, combine aerobic and anaerobic exercise into your routine. Aerobic exercise will really melt the fat off. Anaerobic exercise, such as weight training, will allow you to tone and shape certain areas of your body to create the look that you are after. Think of yourself as a sculptor working with a block of clay. You can use diet and exercise to sculpt the body that you want by chiseling away the fat and toning your muscles to look your best.

Fat-loss strategy #8: Do both aerobic and anaerobic exercise.

FIND A WAY TO MAKE EXERCISE FUN

Exercise should be fun; otherwise, you won't be consistent. —Laura Ramirez

Exercise can and should be fun. It does not have to be drudgery. The key is finding some type of exercise(s) that you enjoy so that you stick with the program. You can also listen to music or books on tape while you walk, run, or whatever. Walking your dog is a great way for both you and your pet to get some exercise.

DO YOU LOVE TO DANCE?

Join a Zumba® class! What's that? Zumba® is supposedly the world's largest and most successful dance fitness program, with millions people of all shapes and sizes taking weekly classes in more than 125 countries. It uses "red-hot international music" and dancing. This is the class for you if you love to dance. Many people who I have spoken with absolutely love this. They say that it is exhilarating and contagious.

Here are some more exercise options for you to consider:

(1) Join a gym.

This is a great option because it gives you access to many different types of fitness equipment. Many gyms offer cardio classes. You have friends and peer support at a gym. It's easier to exercise if everybody around you is exercising. The price of gym memberships has really come down in recent years because of fierce competition among gyms. Pick a gym close to your house or office.

(2) Buy a treadmill.

This is a great option because you can watch

TV, read, study, or baby sit while you exercise. You can also increase the incline on the treadmill as you get into shape. That increases the intensity and burns more calories.

(3) Run outdoors.

If you are really out of shape or more than 30 pound overweight, running will be next to impossible at first. I realize that many people are too heavy and out of condition to run, but if you want fast results and you have the grit and determination, running will melt the fat off of your body faster than any other exercise that I have discovered. Running vacuums the waist like nothing else! If you do decide to run, try to run on soft dirt, on grass, or at the beach. I don't recommend running on hard surfaces. Wearing headphones with your favorite music really helps with the motivation.

(4) Do a combination of walking/running.

Simply run as far as you can until you get tired and then walk for a while. Run some more and then walk some more. This will give you great results fast! You can cover a lot of distance doing this.

(5) Join an aerobics class.

It's sometimes easier to exercise if you have music and peer support with a big group of people. There are many types of aerobic classes. For example, there are step classes, kickboxing classes, and classes that involve using very light weights.

(6) Join a yoga class.

A good friend of mine is a yoga instructor, and she looks amazing.

(7) Go biking outdoors or indoors.

If you live in a rural area or a city with many bike trails, then go for it. Stationary bike classes are very popular at many gyms because they burn a lot of calories in a very short amount of time.

(8) Try Pilates.

Pilates is a conditioning program that emphasizes the balanced development of the body through core strength and flexibility. Core strength is the foundation of Pilates exercise. I tried this, and it was a great workout.

(9) Join a self-defense class.

This will really melt the fat off fast. Have you ever tried hitting a heavy bag for a long period? It's quite a workout.

(10) Go golfing.

The key here is to walk instead of riding in a golf cart!

(11) Work out with a home gym.

This is great if you can afford it and can stay disciplined to work out with all of the distractions.

(12) Walk in the deep sand at the beach.

Enjoy the ocean scenery while you get a great workout. This obviously burns a lot more calories than regular walking.

(13) Take tennis lessons.

This is a good workout and burns a lot of calories. Perhaps invite your workout partner to join you.

(14) Walk in a shopping mall.

Believe it or not, a lot of people do this. It is a safe environment, and you are out of the weather. The key is having the discipline to maintain a fast walking pace and to avoid all of the temptations of the mall.

(15) Swim and/or join a water aerobics class.

This is for people who enjoy being in the water or who might have joint problems.

(16) Circuit train with weights.

This involves training your entire body with weights in one workout with very little rest between sets. You only perform maybe one to two sets per body part. It is a way to turn your weight workout into an aerobic, cardio workout by training very fast with light weights. Never train the same muscle two days in a row. Muscles need at least 48 hours rest between weight workouts. So, maybe attempt this on

Monday, Wednesday, and Friday.

(17) Do a regular workout with weights.

In this case, you should try to exercise each muscle group once per week. For example:

Monday: chest, shoulders, triceps
Tuesday: upper back, biceps, forearms
Thursday: quadriceps and hamstrings
Friday: abdominals, calves, lower back

You take more rest between exercises than with circuit weight training and use heavier weights. You are able to do more sets per body part.

<u>WEIGHT-TRAINING BASICS</u>

WON'T I BECOME "MUSCLE-BOUND" IF I LIFT WEIGHTS?

Some women tell me that they are worried about becoming "muscle-bound" from lifting weights. Women do not have to worry about gaining a lot of muscle like men because women do not have large amounts of testosterone like men do. Women only secrete very tiny amounts of testosterone, so they will not gain a lot of muscle. Women will tone and shape their bodies with a weight-lifting routine. Stick with light weights and do a lot of repetitions to burn calories and tone/sculpt the body that you want. Years ago, gyms were mostly full of men, but nowadays, the gyms are also full of females because women have caught on to the benefits of weight training.

WARM UP

Warming up is critical for any exercise routine, especially weight training. Always do something light and easy before moving on to heavier weights or intense aerobic exercise, to avoid an injury. Start slow and gradually build up the intensity. Make sure the muscles are good and warm before getting into it.

WORK THE BIG MUSCLES BEFORE THE SMALLER MUSCLES

Make sure that you exercise your big muscles before moving on to your smaller muscles. For example, say that you are exercising your upper body by lifting weights at the gym. You want to exercise your relatively large back, chest, and shoulder muscles before exercising your smaller and weaker arm muscles (biceps and triceps). Why is that? Your biceps are heavily involved when working your back muscles. Your triceps are heavily involved when working your chest and shoulder muscles. Those small muscles will tire out long before your bigger muscles. So, fatigue the big muscles first and then move on to the smaller muscles.

STRETCHING

Be sure to do some light stretching to keep yourself limber. I prefer to stretch after my muscles are warm and not before. I believe that there is less chance of injury that way, especially if the weather is cold.

SAMPLE WORKOUT ROUTINES

Obviously, there are a big variety of exercise options available to you. Pick something that you enjoy. Try to exercise for at least 45–60 minutes, five times per week. If you want faster results, exercise more. You can combine different types of exercises to avoid staleness and boredom. Here are a few examples:

Sample workout routine #1:

Monday, Tuesday, Thursday, Friday: weights and cardio machine(s) at the gym

Saturday: walking

Sample workout routine #2:

Monday, Wednesday, Friday: Zumba® class

Saturday: Pilates

Sunday: walk with dog outdoors

Sample workout routine #3:

Monday, Wednesday, Friday: circuit train with weights

Tuesday, Thursday: walk on the incline treadmill

Sample workout routine #4 (a more challenging routine for faster results):

Monday, Wednesday, Friday: weights and cardio machines at the gym

Tuesday, Thursday, Saturday: run/walk outdoors 3–4 miles or more

You get the idea. There is no reason at all that exercise has to be boring. Mix up your routine to avoid hitting a plateau or getting bored. Do what you enjoy so that you stick with the program. Wear headphones if you like music for extra motivation. Start slow and gradually increase the time and intensity of your workouts.

Physical fitness is not only one of the most important keys to a healthy body; it is the basis of dynamic and creative intellectual activity. —John F. Kennedy

CALORIES BURNED PER HOUR FOR VARIOUS ACTIVITIES (FOR A 130 POUND PERSON)

ACTIVITY (CALORIES BURNED)[32]

Aerobics, low impact (295)
Aerobics step (502)
Hiking with pack (413)
Basketball playing (354)
Circuit training (472)
Cycling 9 MPH (472)

Gardening (236)
Golf (carrying clubs) (266)
Handball (708)
Housework moderate (207)
Instructor aerobic (354)
Jumping rope moderate (590)
Kickboxing (590)
Racquetball playing (413)
Running 5 MPH (472)
Stair machine (531)
Stationary cycling vigorous (620)
Stretching yoga (236)
Swimming laps freestyle slow (413)
Tennis singles (472)
Walk/run vigorous (295)
Walk 3 MPH (195)
Walk 3.5 MPH uphill (354)
Water aerobics (236)
Weight lifting vigorous (354)
Weight lifting light (177)

__Fat-loss strategy #9: Gradually work your way up to exercising for at least 45–60 minutes, 5 times per week. Pick exercises that you enjoy so that you stick with the program.__

CHOOSE THE RIGHT EXERCISE PARTNER

If you choose to exercise with a partner who is also trying to lose weight, it can be a good thing because you can feed off of each other's energy. You can motivate and push each other. You are less likely to skip a workout if you know that your training partner is expecting and waiting for you at the gym.

If you are feeling down and unmotivated, your partner can encourage you and lift you up. Conversely, choosing the wrong partner could sap your energy and motivation. It might also help your motivation to hang out with other people who exercise.

Fat-loss strategy #10 : Choose a good exercise partner. You can motivate and push each other.

ADVANCED TRAINING

For those of you who are extra motivated and/or are already in decent condition, I would like to suggest high-intensity interval training (HIIT). I already mentioned HIIT training in the section on boosting your metabolism. To refresh your memory, HIIT involves short, high-intensity bursts of aerobic exercise followed by slow rest periods. Athletes and fitness buffs have used HIIT training for years for very efficient fat loss and conditioning. What are the advantages of HIIT?

(1) It boosts your metabolism for several hours after the workout.

(2) It saves time. You burn a ton of calories in a very short amount of time.

(3) It combats monotony. This is a way to mix up your routine.

(4) It increases your VO2 max (Volume Oxygen Maximum), which is the maximum capacity of an

individual's body to transport and use oxygen during exercise. VO2 max is widely accepted as the single best measure of cardiovascular fitness, and the higher it is, the more fit you are.

(5) It works great for fat loss!

A 2006 study by Jason Talanian and colleagues that was published in the *Journal of Applied Physiology* found that HIIT improves cardio fitness and helps the body to burn more fat. [33] The study involved women riding stationary bikes in hard–easy intervals and found that the women experienced a significant increase in fat burned and aerobic capacity.

HIIT could be used on a stationary bike, stair stepper, treadmill, or elliptical machine, or with walking/running or jumping rope. The possibilities are almost endless. An example of a HITT routine might look like the following:

(1) Warm up for 5 minutes at a very low intensity.

(2) Pick up the pace to an "8" intensity on a "10" scale for 60 seconds.

(3) Slow the pace back down to a "3" intensity for 60 seconds.

(4) Repeat steps 2–3 at least 5 more times.

(5) Cool down for 5 minutes at a "3" intensity.

That's it. Add HIIT into your normal routine a few times per week and speed up your fat-loss results.

BREAKING THROUGH A PLATEAU

Suppose that you seem to have hit a plateau and progress grinds to a halt; what do you do? First of all, make sure that you remember to drop your calories more as you get lighter and lighter. For example, if you drop from 300 pounds down to 250 pounds, you obviously need fewer calories than before. Secondly, be honest with yourself. Have you let your diet and exercise routine slip a bit? Are you eating bigger portions and getting less exercise? Finally, try to mix up your routine and "shock" the body. Our bodies quickly adapt to the stresses that we put on them and become very efficient at certain exercises. For example, if you are always doing the stair machine as part of your exercise routine, certain muscles that you use on the stair machine become much stronger and more efficient. Consequently, you don't have to work as hard as before. Say that you "shock" the body by replacing the stair machine routine with swimming. All of a sudden, you are now using different muscles and the body has to work very hard to try to adapt to the new routine. Before you know it, you have broken through the plateau.

I see beginners come in to the gym all the time and make great progress for the first few months. They do the same weight routine over and over, but after a while, the body adapts to the routine. The muscles are no longer being stressed because they have adapted to the routine. So, progress grinds to a halt. The solution is to mix up the routine and "confuse" the muscles. Do some new exercises that the muscles are not expecting, and progress starts again.

TESTOSTERONE (For men only)

It's a well-known fact that testosterone (T) increases lean body mass (muscle), reduces body fat, and is correlated with libido. It's also well known that obesity reduces T levels in the body and increases an enzyme known as aromatase which converts T into estrogens (female hormones).[34] Increased estrogens in the body are known to further reduce T. This might lead to gynecomastia. Factors known to increase aromatase include age, obesity, smoking, and alcohol.[35] Supplementing with zinc is known to decrease aromatase activity. Lower T in men is also associated with metabolic syndrome, type 2 diabetes, and cardiovascular disease.[36] It becomes a vicious cycle:

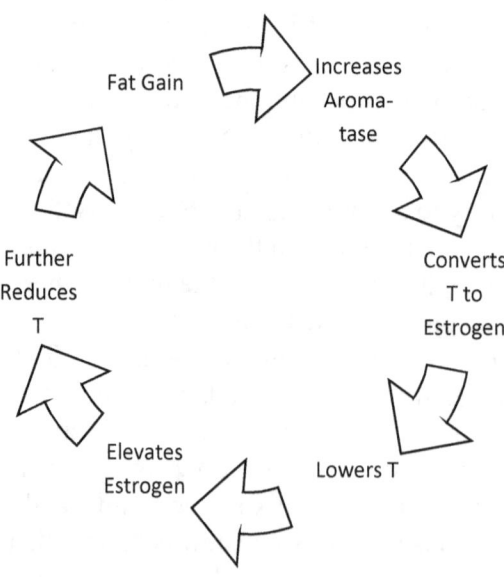

Fat Gain

Increases Aroma- tase

Converts T to Estrogen

Further Reduces T

Lowers T

Elevates Estrogen

So how can we fight back and restore our T levels?

(1) Losing fat--->Reduces aromatase activity--->T goes back to normal

(2) Get enough zinc, which is needed for T production and which decreases aromatase activity.

(3) Eat cruciferous vegetables such as broccoli, cabbage, and Brussels sprouts, which contain phytochemicals called indoles that have been shown to reduce estrogen metabolism.[37]

(4) Go heavy at the gym. Weight training boosts T.

(5) Get enough monounsaturated fat in your diet, which is needed to for the production of T.

(6) Quit smoking and go easy on the alcohol. Remember that smoking and heavy drinking both increase aromatase.

CHAPTER 6:

YOUR SELF-IMAGE AND GETTING MOTIVATED

Just do it! —Nike ™

Some people simply don't believe that it is possible for them to lose weight. It is actually their self-image that is holding them back. Dr. Maxwell Maltz was an American cosmetic surgeon who wrote the best-selling book *Psycho-Cybernetics*, which was published way back in 1960. Dr. Maltz passed away in 1975. The central idea of Dr. Maltz's book is that a person's self-image sets the boundaries of individual accomplishment and defines what he or she can or cannot do. If one's self-image is faulty, all of his efforts will end in failure. The person who conceives himself as a failure will find a way to stay a failure, in spite of his best efforts, willpower, or good intentions. You may have limiting beliefs that are holding you back. Dr. Maltz called the discovery of the self-image the most important psychologic discovery of his century.

Dr. Maltz performed cosmetic surgeries on countless patients with facial deformities and other defects. In most cases, changes in a patient's personality would occur suddenly and dramatically when Dr. Maltz improved the deformity. Usually, the patient would have increased confidence and self-esteem. However, in some cases, the patient had no change after surgery even after Dr. Maltz made their face or other deformity perfect. They kept the same personality and would insist that they looked the same as before even though family and friends would barely recognize them. These patients had a very poor self-image and still saw themselves as "ugly," no matter how handsome or beautiful that they actually looked. It was these cases that intrigued Dr. Maltz.

Each of us has a self-image that has been created from our past experiences, opinions from other people, successes, failures, and beliefs. All of our actions, behaviors, and feelings are consistent with our self-image, and we act like the sort of person that we conceive ourselves to be. Our habits and self-image go together. For example, if a person sees himself as only a "C" student, his beliefs might hold him back from making straight A's. He doesn't think that he has what it takes to make straight A's, so he always finds a way to sabotage himself. It's actually his self-image and beliefs about himself that are holding him back and not his true ability. Likewise, you may have been heavy for years or even for all of your life. You might have a self-image of yourself as a large person. You might have tried countless diets and exercise programs but you have never been able to lose weight. You might have convinced yourself that it is not possible for you. It could actually be a faulty self-image that is holding you back.

The good news is that the self-image can be changed. Change the self-image and you change the personality and behavior. Dr. Maltz recommends using visualization to change the self-image. Visualization affects the subconscious mind. What is visualization? It is the process of creating a mental picture of what you want to happen as if it has already happened. Consistently visualize yourself as thin. What exactly would you look like? How would you feel? What clothes would you be wearing? Visualization is a technique often used by athletes that involves visualizing specific behaviors and events occurring in one's life. Whatever you visualize clearly and often will eventually become part of your reality.

If you think that your self-image may be sabotaging you from losing weight, you may want to try visualization. There is a good reason that Olympic athletes and other high-achievers use visualization: it really works. Visualize reaching your goals in the present tense, as if you have already achieved them. What emotions would you experience? How happy would you be? What size would your waist be? *In your mind, consistently see it, feel it, experience it, and live it. Once you get in the habit of regularly visualizing yourself as thin, you will find that your doubts begin to disappear, and your enthusiasm increases.*

THE NEW YEAR'S PEOPLE

Being defeated is often a temporary condition. Giving up is what makes it permanent. —Marilyn Vos Savant

I work out regularly at the local gym. Every January, there is a huge surge in memberships at my gym and gyms across America due to people making their New Year's resolutions to finally exercise, eat right, lose weight, and get into shape. By February, the crowd has died down a bit, and by March, the New Year's crowd is gone. All that remains are the regulars. If those New Year's people did lose any weight, it's all going to come back after they return to their unhealthy diets and quit exercising.

What happened to the New Year's people? They started off with good intentions, high hopes, and new goals, but somewhere along the way, they lost their motivation, gave up, and threw in the towel. I am here to help you get and keep that motivation. Are you going to be one of the New Year's people who gives up easily and quits, or are you going to reach your goals?

PERSISTENCE

Energy and persistence conquer all things. —Benjamin Franklin

If you throw in the towel like the New Year's people and give up easily, your failure rate is guaranteed to be 100%. Nobody said that it was going to be easy. If you persist long enough, you will eventually reach your goals. I will tell you right now that you need to maintain the healthy lifestyle if you want to keep the weight off. Going back to your old ways means gaining all of the fat back that you worked so hard to get rid of. I assume that your ultimate goal is good health and not just weight loss. Doesn't everybody want good health? Consider that every time you eat a healthy meal or get through a workout, you are moving one step closer to your ultimate goal of good health.

OTHER PEOPLE SIMPLY CAN'T GET MOTIVATED

It seems to me that a lot of people know that they should be eating right and exercising to lose weight, but they just can't seem to get motivated. Maybe they don't want to cut down on the unhealthy foods, or they keep putting it off because they say that they are too busy or have countless other excuses. It's time to quit making excuses and get to work.

We can accomplish almost anything if we have enough motivation. Skeptical? If somebody offered you $10 million to reach your goal weight within two years or less, you would find a way to do it, wouldn't you? I am betting that you would. I'm betting that you would reach your goal weight in record time! That's the power of motivation. Well, the bad news is that nobody is going to offer you $10 million, but what is your good health worth to you? For me, it is priceless. If your motivation is strong enough, you will find a way to lose weight and keep it off.

Fat-loss strategy #11: A big key to losing weight and keeping it off is finding a way to fuel your motivation.

If you are overweight, you are putting yourself at risk for a host of health problems, especially type 2 diabetes.[38]

The following information is from the American Diabetes Association:

* 80% of type 2 diabetes cases are related to obesity.

* Type 2 diabetes accounts for 90–95% of all cases of diabetes.

* 25.8 million children and adults in the United States have diabetes.

* 79 million Americans have prediabetes (35% of adults in US).

Type 2 diabetes has become a huge epidemic in the US. The following chart shows how cases have exploded since 1980:

Type 2 Diabetes Cases (US)

Source: American Diabetes Association

In order to change we must be sick and tired of being sick and tired. —*Anonymous*

CALCULATING YOUR BODY MASS INDEX (BMI)

Your BMI is a better measure of your weight than simply weighing yourself on a scale because it takes into account your height as well. The BMI applies to most of the population. However, the BMI formula has limitations. The BMI formula does not apply to many athletes and other people who are carrying a lot of muscle. For example, a typical linebacker in the National Football League might be 6' 2" tall and weigh 240 pounds. He represents somebody who is in peak physical condition. According to the BMI formula, this linebacker would be considered obese. But for somebody who is not carrying a lot of muscle, a very high BMI correlates with obesity and type 2 diabetes. So, hopefully, this will help motivate you to shed some pounds.

Here is the formula:

BMI = (weight pounds x 703)/(height inches x height inches)

1. Multiply your weight in pounds by 703.

2. Multiply your height in inches by itself (height x height).

3. Divide line 1 by line 2 to get BMI.

BMI Categories:

Under 25 = Normal weight
25 to 29 = Overweight
30 and above = Obese

My fat scares me—it's a ticking time bomb. —*Carrie Latet*

TRANSITION INTO A HEALTHY LIFESTYLE SLOWLY

If you are really out of shape and have a horrible diet, it might be very tough to go full throttle into an exercise routine and healthy diet, so I recommend that you start slowly. Maybe aim for a 30-minute workout just three times per week at first. Gradually add time and intensity to your workouts. Eventually work your way up to 45–60 minutes of exercise, at least five days/week. I think that a lot of people quit and give up if the exercise is too long or difficult at first. Gradually get into shape. The good news is that exercise becomes much easier as you slowly get into shape. Your heart, lungs, and muscles become much stronger and more efficient. As the fat melts off, you are carrying less weight around. Believe it or not, you will get to the point where you no longer dread your workouts and actually look forward to working out. Once you are in shape, you feel like you are on top of the world and like you could run forever. Believe me; it's worth all of the hard work. So, how do we get motivated and stay motivated?

FOCUS ON THE REWARDS OF
SUCCESSFULLY LOSING WEIGHT

I want you to write down every possible reason that you can think of to lose weight. Make a list. The idea is to give yourself enough motivation to deal with a strict diet and exercise. Here are some ideas to get you started:

(1) Improve your health.

(2) Improve your sex life.

(3) Feel more attractive.

(4) Be able to do activities without getting exhausted.

(5) Get compliments on how good you are looking.

(6) Look good at your high school reunion.

(7) Look great in and out of clothes.

(8) Be able to go out and buy a new wardrobe.

(9) Get the beach body that you always wanted.

(10) Look 10 years younger.

(11) Boost your energy.

(12) Be around to enjoy your grandchildren.

(13) Run a marathon, or at least make it up a flight of

stairs without getting winded.

(14) Feel 10 years younger.

Only you can figure out what motivates you. Make a list and keep it in front of you daily. When the going gets tough, focus on the rewards of successfully losing weight. It will get you through those tough workouts.

REWARD YOURSELF FOR LOSING WEIGHT—YOU DESERVE IT!

Say that your big goal is to shed 50 pounds. Set smaller goals along the way and reward yourself for reaching those smaller goals. For example, a reasonable goal might be to lose two pounds per week. If after four weeks, you have lost eight pounds, reward yourself with something like getting a massage or a new music CD. Once you have shed the entire 50 pounds, reward yourself with a new wardrobe and/or a vacation. You deserve it. Just be sure to maintain a reasonably healthy diet while on vacation. Needless to say, try to reward yourself with something other than fattening food. Possibly create a rewards list and keep it hanging someplace that you will see it daily. Anything for some extra motivation!

Fat-loss strategy #12: Set weight goals and persist.

Patience, persistence, and perspiration make an unbeatable combination for success. —Napoleon Hill

KEEP A FOOD JOURNAL

Keeping a food journal is a great idea because you can get a general sense of how many calories you are actually consuming each day. Record every little snack and drink so you can see where the calories are really coming from. You might just be surprised. You can look up the calories on the food lists that I provided in chapter 3, on food labels, in a book, or in an online database. You can also record your emotions and figure out if you eat because you are actually hungry or simply because you are bored, depressed, stressed, or whatever. Some people may overeat at certain times or in certain places or with certain people. Be sure to record portion sizes and also drinks.

As I already mentioned in the introduction, you should see a doctor and record your blood pressure, cholesterol, blood sugar, C-reactive protein, triglycerides, and resting heart rate. Record these numbers in your journal. Watching these numbers improve as you start to eat right and exercise can be very motivating. You might also want to have pictures taken of yourself and to record your body measurements in your journal for extra motivation.

Fat-loss strategy #13: Keep a food journal.

MOTIVATIONAL MUSIC

I frequently go out and run beneath the beautiful Sandia Mountains in Albuquerque. I am usually very motivated, but I must admit that there

are some days when the motivation is lacking. Once I put on my headphones with some motivational music, my lazy attitude quickly changes. Good music energizes and motivates me. It makes it so much easier to get through a tough workout. If you are a music lover like me, I highly recommend that you invest in a music player if you don't already have one and load it full of your favorite motivational music. It will help you get through those tough workouts.

CHAPTER 7:

KEEPING THE WEIGHT OFF

Most people fail, not because of lack of desire, but because of lack of commitment. —Vince Lombardi

In this chapter, we explore the characteristics of people who have successfully lost weight and kept it off, and I give an example of somebody who makes use of all the strategies in this book to lose fat.

THE NATIONAL WEIGHT CONTROL REGISTRY

The National Weight Control Registry (NWCR) was established in 1994. It was developed to identify and investigate the characteristics of individuals who have succeeded at long-term weight loss. It is currently tracking over 10,000 individuals who have lost significant amounts of weight and kept it off for long periods of time. Registry members have lost an average of 66 pounds and kept it off for 5.5 years.[39] Here are some key findings of the NWCR:

* 98% of Registry participants modified their food intake in some way to lose weight.

* 94% increased their physical activity, with the most frequently reported form of activity being walking.

* 78% eat breakfast every day, and 90% reported eating breakfast at least five days per week.

* 75% weigh themselves at least once per week.

* 62% watch less than 10 hours of TV per week.

* 90% exercise, on average, about one hour per day.

Notice that 78% of the successful weight-loss individuals eat breakfast every day. People sometimes skip breakfast thinking that they are cutting calories, but by midmorning that person is starved. Breakfast skippers end up binging throughout the day and set themselves up for failure.

Fat-loss strategy #14: Eat breakfast every day.

Maybe you will join the NWCR once you have lost the weight and kept if off for a long period of time?

WATCH OUT FOR THE FAD DIETS

There is nothing magical about successfully losing weight. You have got to do it by cutting calories and exercising. Unfortunately, there are a lot of fad diets and gimmicks out there that promise miraculous results quickly. Here are some signs of a fad diet:

(1) It promises a quick and effortless fix.

(2) It sounds too good to be true.

(3) It restricts or eliminates healthy fat or good carbs. "People need to wake up to the reality that diets that restrict entire food groups—especially essential carbohydrates like fruits and vegetables—are unhealthy and can be dangerous," says former Surgeon General C. Everett Koop, founder of Shape Up America! These types of diets might put your body in a state of ketosis and you might end up being fatigued, dizzy, weak, and lethargic. Healthy fat is not the enemy and neither are good carbs. You might be able to temporarily lose weight on a very low-carb or fat-free diet. However, the weight loss is actually from cutting calories. Those types of diets are not sustainable over the long haul. You need healthy carbs and a reasonable amount of fat in your diet for good health.

(4) It claims that weight can be lost and maintained with little or no exercise. Notice that 90% of the successful weight losers on the National Weight Control Registry exercise for an hour per day on average.

(5) It advocates losing more than two to three pounds per week. Unless you are extremely obese, losing more than that is not realistic or healthy.

(6) It is a detox diet. This diet can't be maintained, and any weight that you might lose comes right back.

(7) It is the eat-all-you-want diet. The theory here is

that you gorge on your favorite foods until you become sick of them and no longer crave the bad foods. Wouldn't it be great if it was that easy? Unfortunately, this plan falls flat. You gain a ton of weight and eventually crave the bad food again.

PUTTING IT ALL TOGETHER

Mike is age 45 and weighs 260 pounds at 5' 10". He wants to get down to 170 pounds, but he has been overweight most of his life and does not think that it is possible for him to lose weight. He has tried many fad diets in the past, but nothing has worked for him. He usually has very low energy, watches six hours of TV daily, and gets very little exercise. Mike frequently skips breakfast or has half a pound of bacon, whole eggs cooked in butter, and a pot of coffee. His lunch consists of a super-size double cheeseburger, fries, and a soda from the local burger joint. Dinner is pizza with extra cheese and whole milk. He snacks on ice cream and salty chips, and drinks several sodas per day. He does not sleep well due to his caffeine addiction and sleep apnea. His blood sugar shoots up and down, which causes wild mood swings. After Mike's best friend has a heart attack at age 50, Mike decides to go to the doctor and get checked out. Mike discovers that he has high blood pressure, extremely high LDL cholesterol, and prediabetes. Mike's triglycerides are also sky-high from his high-fructose diet, which explains his leptin resistance and constant hunger. His doctor advises him to diet, exercise, and lose weight. Mike has been slowly gaining weight for years and currently eats 2,600–3,000 calories per day, which mostly come from fast food and high-calorie snacks at home.

Mike's doctor warns that medications may be necessary if Mike can't get his weight under control.

Mike decides that it is time for a change. His life depends on it. The triggering event for Mike is his friend's heart attack. He decides to exercise three to five days per week and determines that he should cut his food intake down to around 1,600 calories per day to safely lose two pounds of fat per week. He begins by walking three days per week. At first, he can barely do a mile without getting exhausted and winded because he is so out of shape. He begins eating breakfast, which now consists of egg whites, oatmeal, and a slice of 100% whole-wheat toast with honey. He replaces the double cheeseburger with a turkey sandwich and salad. He replaces the pizza and whole milk with grilled salmon, vegetables, and 1%-fat milk. Instead of snacking on ice cream, he snacks on fat-free frozen yogurt and frozen grapes. He still has a big sweet-tooth, so he snacks on sweet fruits like oranges and strawberries. Instead of drinking a six-pack of sugary soda daily, he now drinks many glasses of filtered water daily, which satisfies his thirst and dulls any hunger pangs that he may have. Mike replaces the white bread in his diet with 100% whole-wheat bread and replaces the bacon, sausage, and processed lunch meats with lean chicken tenderloins, tuna, wild salmon, and organic, grass-fed, lean beef.

Mike struggles at first, but then he begins to notice changes. He falls asleep faster and sleeps better because of the exercise and reduced caffeine consumption. His energy begins to increase because he got rid of all the processed sugar foods and cut his sodium intake down from 4,000 mg daily to less than 1,500 mg daily. He replaces the salty chips with plain popcorn, and his blood pressure begins to drop. He begins to slowly lose weight. He increases his walking from one mile per day up to two miles per day, four days per week. Mike replaces the saturated and trans fat in his diet with healthy fat from nuts, seeds, fish, and healthy oils. Instead of cooking with lard or butter, he now uses canola oil. Instead of smothering his salads with fatty, salty dressings, he uses a small amount of olive oil. His bad LDL cholesterol levels begin to drop. The plaque in his arteries begins to clear out. He cuts the processed foods from his diet and loads up on fruits and vegetables. Mike is now losing two pounds of fat per week.

A little more persistence, a little more effort, and what seemed hopeless failure may turn to glorious success. —Elbert Hubbard

After 16 weeks, Mike has shed 32 pounds of fat. He begins getting compliments from friends and family on how much better he is looking. They want to know his secret. Mike feels so much better. He sleeps better, has more energy, and does not have wild mood swings anymore. He gets an emotional lift from the exercise. Mike begins to add some circuit weight training to his exercise routine. His heart and lung function have improved and he begins to slowly add running to his walking regimen. He increases his daily distance to three miles. He now runs/walks three days per week and circuit weight trains two days per week at the gym. Mike cuts his daily calories even more since he is now 32 pounds lighter. Mike saves money because he is eating less food in general and less restaurant food.

After 40 weeks, Mike has lost 80 pounds of fat and reached his target weight of 170 pounds. He has reached his goal in less than one year. All of the hard work has paid off. He rewards himself with a new wardrobe and a vacation to Hawaii. He deserves it. Mike's friends and family barely recognize him anymore. He looks and feels 10 years younger. He is full of energy. His sleep apnea is gone, and he now sleeps great every night. Mike goes back to the doctor for his annual checkup, and the doctor is astounded. Mike's blood pressure is down to normal. His cholesterol levels are now normal, and he no longer has prediabetes. Mike's triglyceride levels have plummeted, which has cleared up his leptin resistance. Therefore, the natural leptin in his body is now reaching his brain, and he no longer experiences extreme hunger. His resting heart rate has dropped significantly, which is a sign of improved fitness. Mike maintains his weight loss because he continues a healthy lifestyle.

MAINTAIN A HEALTHY LIFESTYLE TO KEEP THE WEIGHT OFF

Motivation is what gets you started. Habit is what keeps you going. —Jim Rohn

Some people lose weight and then eventually gain it all back and then some. Why? It's from crash dieting and losing the weight too quickly, giving up the exercise routine, or from fad diets that are difficult to stick with. For example, if your diet is too restrictive, you may stick with it for a while, but you may eventually give in to your cravings and quit the diet. The answer is moderation. Have that occasional bowl of ice cream, but don't make it a daily habit. Some people think that just because they lost the weight, they can go back to their old ways that made them gain weight in the first place. Nothing could be further from the truth. You have to maintain the healthy lifestyle if you want to keep the weight off. That means getting enough exercise and avoiding the empty-calorie carbs and calorie-dense, saturated-fat foods as much as possible.

Fat-loss strategy #15: Maintain a healthy lifestyle once you have lost the weight, to keep it off.

A FINAL WORD

Dreams seldom materialize on their own. — Dian Fossey

I have given you a blueprint and all of the tools necessary to shed fat and get the body that you want. All of the work is up to you. There is no quick and easy way to shed a lot of fat. Hopefully, I have convinced you that eating healthy, cutting calories, and exercising is the way to go. It takes hard work, persistence, and dedication. Over time, I know that you can do it. You have read this far. That tells me that you are serious about losing weight and getting into shape. Just thinking about it and talking about it is not enough to make it happen. You have got to get to work. That means exercising regularly and eating smart. Losing weight is not just about looking great—it's about feeling good and having excellent health. Every healthy meal and every workout moves you one step closer to your goal. Conversely, every time that you eat junk or skip a workout, that moves you further away from your goal. You can give up easily and throw in the towel, or you can get to work and make it happen. It's up to you. Commit to a healthy lifestyle to shed the fat and keep it off. Get started today.

He who hesitates is lost. —Proverb

QUESTIONS AND ANSWERS

What if I simply can't avoid empty-calorie junk food?

Moderation is the key. Have an occasional treat, but don't make junk food the centerpiece of your diet.

How do I handle cravings?

Remember that you can gorge on fruits and vegetables all day long and consume very few calories. It's the high-density foods that cause the weight gain. Substitute healthy, low-calorie foods for junk food. Here are some examples:

* Replace ice cream with sugar-free frozen yogurt or frozen grapes.

* Replace candy with sweet fruits such as strawberries.

* Replace those high-calorie, salty chips with plain popcorn.

* Replace the sugary colas with filtered water and a lemon slice, which helps to fill you up. If you think that you are feeling hungry, try drinking some water, and then wait 10–15 minutes and reevaluate.

How much weight should I try to lose each week?

Aim for 1–2 pounds per week. That might not

seem like much, but over six months, that is 26–52 pounds, which is very realistic and healthy. Remember that if you lose weight faster than that, you are likely losing a lot of muscle along with the fat unless you are extremely obese.

Is exercising just one or two times per week enough?

No, not really. It's better than nothing, but if you want to see significant results, aim for at least five times per week.

But, but, but, I don't have time to exercise. What can I do?

Make your health a priority. No excuses. The 30–60 minutes of daily exercise does not have to be done all at once. You could do a quick 15-minute workout in the morning before work and then walk around your office parking lot at lunch break for 30 minutes. How about buying a treadmill and setting it up in front of the TV? You can watch TV/read/study while you exercise.

I go to the gym but don't see any results. What can I do?

Be honest with yourself. Are you actually working out, or are you spending most of your time socializing and bobbing up and down in the pool? Working your jaw muscles does not count as exercise. All kidding aside, you really need to put some intensity into your workouts and work up a good sweat. Challenge yourself. Also, remember to cut calories for weight loss.

Should I try to sweat the weight off with a special weight-loss plastic suit?

No. That could actually be dangerous, and you might overheat. You will only lose a lot of water and gain it all back as soon as you replenish the water you lost.

All of my favorite foods are on the empty-calorie list or full of saturated fat. What can I do?

That's why you gained weight in the first place. The key is moderation. Have some occasional junk food, but don't make it the main course in your diet.

I exercise and eat healthy, but I am still not losing weight. What am I doing wrong?

Even healthy food has calories. You have to cut calories. Cut your daily food intake by 500–1,000 calories and continue to exercise.

I lose weight and then gain it all back. What can I do?

Maintain a healthy lifestyle. Just because you lost the weight, that's no excuse to fall off the wagon and go back to your old ways.

I get bored when I exercise. What can I do?

Listen to music. Wear headphones with your favorite, motivational music. Exercise with a friend.

How do I stick with an exercise routine?

Find something that you enjoy. Find an exercise partner. You are less likely to skip a workout if you know that your partner is at the gym waiting for you and is depending on you to help keep him/her motivated.

Should I cut sodium intake to zero?

No, unless advised by a physician. That could actually be dangerous, especially if you sweat a lot. Hyponatremia can occur if the body gets too low in sodium. This can happen in athletes that sweat a lot, since sodium is lost through perspiration. Our bodies need a very small amount of sodium, but most Americans consume way too much.

Could I lose weight by consuming only 1,000 calories per day from diet candy bars?

Technically, yes you could. However, you would soon crash and burn because our bodies need a balanced amount of proteins, carbohydrates, fats, vitamins, minerals, fiber, and water to be healthy.

You would soon develop vitamin and mineral deficiencies, for example. That's also why a total starvation diet won't work either. We need daily nutrients to keep our bodies healthy and functioning properly. Also, a total starvation diet would cause our bodies to go into "famine mode," and our metabolisms would drastically slow down. So a key to successful weight loss is a well-balanced diet.

I am very interested in supplementing with L-arginine. Where can I find more information?

I recommend reading the book *NO More Heart Disease* by Dr. Louis J. Ignarro.

SUMMARY OF THE FAT-LOSS STRATEGIES

Fat-loss strategy #1: Reduce calories for weight loss, but also eat a nutritious, well-balanced diet.

Fat-loss strategy #2: Cut down on processed carbohydrates, especially refined fructose. Make every calorie count.

Fat-loss strategy #3: Cut down on saturated fat foods. Totally eliminate trans fat from your diet.

Fat-loss strategy #4: Minimize processed foods as much as possible. Focus on eating wholesome, natural foods in their natural state and in proper amounts.

Fat-loss strategy #5: Minimize sodium in your diet.

Fat-loss strategy #6: Drink several glasses of filtered water every day. Replace sugary colas and other high-calorie drinks with filtered water. Water will fill you up when you feel hungry and it has zero calories.

Fat-loss strategy #7: Women who weigh less than 250 pounds should aim for 1,200 calories/day. Men who weigh less than 250 pounds should aim for 1,400 calories/day. Both men and women who weigh 250–300 pounds should aim for 1,600 calories/day. Both men and women who weigh over 300 pounds should aim for 1,800 calories/day.

Fat-loss strategy #8: Do both aerobic and anaerobic exercise.

Fat-loss strategy #9: Gradually work your way up to exercising for at least 45–60 minutes, five times per week. Pick exercises that you enjoy so that you stick with the program.

Fat-loss strategy #10: Choose a good exercise partner. You can motivate and push each other.

Fat-loss strategy #11: A big key to losing weight and keeping it off is finding a way to fuel your motivation.

Fat-loss strategy #12: Set weight goals and persist.

Fat-loss strategy #13: Keep a food journal.

Fat-loss strategy #14: Eat breakfast every day.

Fat-loss strategy #15: Maintain a healthy lifestyle once you have lost the weight, to keep it off.

REFERENCES

1. Jia Haomiao, et al., "Trends in Quality-Adjusted Life- Years Lost Contributed by Smoking and Obesity," *American Journal of Preventative Medicine*, Volume (February 2010), Issue 2, pp. 138-144.

2. Rideout VJ, Foehr UG, Roberts DF, "Generation of M2 Media in the Lives of 8-18 Year Olds," *A Kaiser Family Foundation Study* (2010).

3. Curtis Michael, "The Obesity Epidemic in the Pacific Islands," *Journal of Development and Social Transformation*, (2010). http://www.maxwell.syr.edu/uploadedFiles/moynihan /dst/curtis5.pdf?n=3228

4. Kovacs Jenny, "Diets of the World: The Japanese Diet," *WebMD*, (2009). http://www.webmd.com/diet/features/diets-of-world-japanese-diet

5. Sacks Frank, et al., "Comparison of weight-loss

diets with different compositions of fat, protein, and carbohydrates," *The New England Journal of Medicine,* (February 26, 2009). http://www.nejm.org/doi/full/10.1056/NEJMoa08047 48

6. Ingalls AM, "Obese, a new mutation in the house mouse," *J. Hered.* 41, (December 1950), (12): pp. 317–8.

7. Considine RV, et al., "Serum immunoreactive-leptin concentrations in normal-weight and obese humans," *N. Engl. J. Med.,* 334, (February 1996), (5): pp. 292–295. http://www.nejm.org/doi/full/10.1056/NEJM1996020 13340503

8. Wang J, et al., "Overfeeding rapidly induces leptin and insulin resistance," *Diabetes,* (December 2001), 50 (12): pp. 2786–2791. http://diabetes.diabetesjournals.org/content/50/12/278 6

9. Enriori PJ, et al., "Diet-induced obesity causes severe but reversible leptin resistance in arcuate melanocortin neurons," *Cell Metab.* 5 (March 2007), (3): pp. 181–194.   http://www.cell.com/cell-metabolism/retrieve/pii/S1550413107000368

10. Banks WA, et al.,"Triglycerides Induce Leptin Resistance at the Blood-Brain Barrier," *Diabetes,* vol.53 no. 5, (May 2004), pp. 1253-1260. http://diabetes.diabetesjournals.org/content/53/5/1253

.full

11. Putnam J., "Food consumption, prices, and expenditures 1970–91," *Economic Research Service*, (1999), Washington, DC: US Department of Agriculture.

12. Teff KL, et al., "Dietary fructose reduces circulating insulin and leptin, attentuates postrandial suppression of ghrelin, and increases triglycerides in women," *The Journal of Clinical Endocrinology & Metabolism*, vol. 89 no. 6 (June 1, 2004), pp. 2963-2972. http://jcem.endojournals.org/content/89/6/2963.abstract

13. Shapiro John, et al., "Fructose-Induced Leptin Resistance Exacerbates Weight Gain in Response to Subsequent High Fat Feeding," *AJP Regulatory Integrative and Comparative Physiology,* (October, 2008). http://ajpregu.physiology.org/content/295/5/R1370

14. Kirschmann John and Dunne Lavon, *Nutrition Almanac (second edition),* McGraw-Hill, (1984) p.5.

15. Mendosa David, "Revised International Table of Glycemic Index (GL) and Glycemic Load (GL) Values-2008," *Mendosa.com*, (2008). http://www.mendosa.com/gilists.htm

16. "Glycemic Index and Diabetes," by the American Diabetes Association/Food & Fitness, (2012). http://www.diabetes.org/food-and-

fitness/food/planning-meals/glycemic-index-and-diabetes.html

17. "Transforming the Food Supply: Report of the Trans Fat Task Force," by Health Canada, (June 2006). http://www.hc-sc.gc.ca/fn-an/nutrition/gras-trans-fats/tf-ge/tf-gt_rep-rap-eng.php

18. Lopez-Garcia E, et al., "Consumption of trans fatty acids is related to plasma biomarkers of inflammation and endothelial dysfunction," *J Nutr*, 135(3): (March 2005), pp. 62-6. http://jn.nutrition.org/content/135/3/562.full.pdf

19. Pradhan AD, et al., "C-reactive protein, interleukin 6, and risk of developing type 2 diabetes mellitus," *JAMA* 286 (3), (2001), pp. 327–34. http://jama.ama-assn.org/content/286/3/327

20. Sijbrands EJ, et al., "Genetic variation, C-reactive protein levels, and incidence of diabetes," *Diabetes,* (March 2007), 56 (3): pp. 872–8. http://diabetes.diabetesjournals.org/content/56/3/872.full.pdf

21. "How can I lower cholesterol," by the American Heart Association, (2007). http://www.heart.org/idc/groups/heart-public/@wcm/@hcm/documents/downloadable/ucm_300460.pdf

22. "Propylene glycol," by Wikipedia, (2012).

http://en.wikipedia.org/wiki/Propylene_glycol

23. "Jack LaLanne Fit As Ever at 70," by the Lodi News-Sentinel, UPI. , (19 November 1984), Retrieved 24 January 2011.

24. "Dietary reference intakes for water, potassium, sodium, chloride, and sulfate," by the Institute of Medicine. 1st ed. Washington, DC: The National Academics Press; (2004).

25. "Most Americans Should Consume Less Sodium," By the Centers for Disease Control and Prevention/SALT HOME (online), (2012). http://www.cdc.gov/salt/

26. "Polyunsaturated Fat," by Wikipedia, (2012). http://en.wikipedia.org/wiki/Polyunsaturated_fat

27. Malaguarnera M, et al., "L-carnitine supplementation reduces oxidized LDL cholesterol in patients with diabetes," *The American Journal of Clinical Nutrition*, vol. 89 no. 1, (January 2007), pp. 71-76. http://www.ajcn.org/content/89/1/71.full

28. Dulloo AG, et al., "Efficacy of a green tea extract rich in catechin polyphenols and caffeine in increasing 24-h energy expenditure and fat oxidation in humans," *Am. J.   Clin. Nutr.* 70, (1999), (6): pp. 1040–5.

29. Lucotti P, et al.,"Beneficial effects of long-term oral L-arginine treatment added to a hypocaloric diet

and exercise training program in obese, insulin resistant diabetic   patients," *The American Journal of Physiology*, (2006). http://ajpendo.physiology.org/content/291/5/E906.full.pdf

30. "Basal Metabolic Rate," by Wikipedia, (2012). http://en.wikipedia.org/wiki/Basal_metabolic_rate

31. Ferraro R, et al., "Lower sedentary metabolic rate in women compared with men," *J Clin Invest.*, (1992 Sep), 90(3): pp. 780-4.

32. "Calories burned during exercise," by Nutri Strategy (online). http://www.nutristrategy.com/activitylist4.htm

33. Talanian Jason, et al., "Two weeks of high-intensity aerobic interval training increases the capacity for fat oxidation during exercise in women," *Journal of Applied   Physiology*, (Sept 26, 2006). http://jap.physiology.org/content/102/4/1439.short

34. Cohen PG, "Obesity in men: the hypogonadal-estrogen receptor relationship and its effects on glucose homeostasis," *Med Hypotheses*, 70(2), (2007 Sep 6), pp. 358-60. http://www.ncbi.nlm.nih.gov/pubmed/17825496

35. "Aromatase," by Wikipedia, (2012). http://en.wikipedia.org/wiki/Aromatase

36. Miner MM, et al., "Testosterone and aging: What have we learned since the Institute of Medicine Report and what lies ahead?" *International Journal of Clinical Practice* posted (05/21/2007), *Int J Clin Pract,* (2007), 61(4): pp. 622-632.
http://www.medscape.com/viewarticle/556617

37. Telang NT, et al., "Inhibition of proliferation and modulation of estradiol metabolism: novel mechanisms for breast cancer prevention by the phytochemical indole-3-carbinol," *Proceedings of the Society for Experimental Biology and Medicine,* (1997), 216: pp. 246-252.

38. "Clinical Guidelines on the Identification, Evaluation, and Treatment of Overweight and Obesity in Adults," by the NIH, NHLBI Obesity Education Initiative, (2012).
http://www.nhlbi.nih.gov/guidelines/obesity/ob_gdln s.pdf

39. "NWCR Facts," by the National Weight Control Registry, Brown Medical School/The Mirian Hospital Weight Control & Diabetes Research Center, (2012).
http://www.nwcr.ws/Research/default.htm

ABOUT THE AUTHOR

Eddie E. Erickson has 33 years of bodybuilding and powerlifting experience and has worked as a personal trainer. In addition to successfully losing a lot of weight himself and keeping it off, he has helped others to reach their weight loss and fitness goals. He trades stock options and is owner of Erickson Enterprises LLC. He has degree in Computer Programming from the University of New Mexico and currently lives in Albuquerque.